PARENTAL ALIENATION, DSM-5, AND ICD-11

D1716170

Publication Number 1113

AMERICAN SERIES
IN
BEHAVIORAL SCIENCE AND LAW

Edited by

RALPH SLOVENKO, B.E., LL.B., M.A., Ph.D.

Professor of Law and Psychiatry
Wayne State University Law School
Detroit, Michigan

PARENTAL ALIENATION, DSM-5, AND ICD-11

Edited by

WILLIAM BERNET, M.D.

Professor, Department of Psychiatry
Vanderbilt University School of Medicine
Nashville, Tennessee

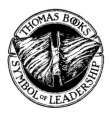

CHARLES C THOMAS · PUBLISHER, LTD.
Springfield · Illinois · U.S.A.

Published and Distributed Throughout the World by

CHARLES C THOMAS • PUBLISHER, LTD.
2600 South First Street
Springfield, Illinois 62794-9265

© 2010 by CHARLES C THOMAS • PUBLISHER, LTD.

ISBN 978-0-398-07944-4 (hard)
ISBN 978-0-398-07945-1 (paper)

Library of Congress Catalog Card Number: 2010012349

With THOMAS BOOKS *careful attention is given to all details of manufacturing
and design. It is the Publisher's desire to present books that are satisfactory as to their
physical qualities and artistic possibilities and appropriate for their particular use.*
THOMAS BOOKS *will be true to those laws of quality that assure a good name
and good will.*

Printed in the United States of America
MM-R-3

Library of Congress Cataloging in Publication Data

Parental alienation, DSM-5, and ICD-11 / edited by William Bernet.
    p. cm.
"Publication Number 1113"–Ser. t.p.
Includes biographical references and index.
ISBN 978-0-398-07944-4 (hard)–ISBN 978-0-398-07945-1 (pbk.)
1. Parental alienation syndrome–Diagnosis. 2. Parental alienation syndrome–Classification. 3. Diagnostic and statistical manual of mental disorders. 5th ed. 4. International statistical classification of diseases and related
health problems. 11th revision. I. Bernet, William. II. Series: American
series in behavioral science and law.
[DNLM: 1. Diagnostic and Statistical Manual of Mental Disorders.
2. International Classification of Diseases. 3. Mental Disorders–classification. 4. Child Custody. 5. International Classification of Diseases. 6. Parent-
Child Relations. 7. Psychiatric Status Rating Scales. 8. Syndrome. WM 15
P228 2010]

RJ506.P27P37 2010
618.92'89–dc22   2010012349

CONTENTS

CONTRIBUTORS

This document was developed by a large number of mental health professionals, legal professionals, and other interested individuals. Many people contributed sections of the text and citations for the bibliography. While this is a consensus document, it should not be assumed that every contributor agrees with every statement made in this book. Also, the agencies and institutions mentioned here are for the purpose of providing each contributor's affiliations; it should not be inferred that each agency and institution officially endorses our proposal that parental alienation be included in DSM-5 and ICD-11.

José M. Aguilar, Ph.D., a forensic psychologist who practices in Córdoba, Spain, has studied parental alienation in Spain. He published books on this topic, lectured extensively, and worked with an agency, Ombudsman for Children of Madrid.

Katherine Andre, Ph.D., is a clinical and forensic psychologist who practices in Northern California. She has been a chairperson for a county Mental Health Board and is currently a professional advisor for a Depression and Bipolar Support Chapter.

E. James Anthony, M.D., a child and adolescent psychiatrist and psychoanalyst, studied the phenomenon of *folie à deux*. He is a former president of the American Academy of Child and Adolescent Psychiatry.

Mila Arch Marin, Ph.D., is a professor at the University of Barcelona. She is an expert in forensic psychology and has written about parental alienation and DSM-5.

Eduard Bakalář, C.Sc., a psychologist who practices in Prague, Czech Republic, has studied parental alienation in the Czech Republic.

Amy J. L. Baker, Ph.D., a psychologist in New York, New York, has conducted research on adult survivors of parental alienation. Dr. Baker is the director of reseach at the Vincent J. Fontana Center for Child Protection.

Paul Bensussan, M.D., is a National Psychiatric Expert appointed by the Cour de cassation (the French Supreme Court). He has been a member of the commission of specialists for the Ministry of Justice, dealing with false allegations of sexual abuse during parental separation and divorce. Dr. Bensussan regularly speaks on these topics at the National School of Magistracy, which trains judges in France.

Alice C. Bernet, M.S.N., is a psychiatric nurse practitioner. She is a graduate student at Vanderbilt University School of Nursing.

Kristin Bernet, M.L.I.S., a research librarian who works in Washington, D.C., is a distance education librarian and an instructor in information literacy at The Johns Hopkins University Washington Library Resource Center.

Barry S. Bien, L.L.B., is a family law attorney in Amherstview, Ontario, who specializes in issues of custody, access, and parental alienation.

Wilfrid von Boch-Galhau, M.D., a psychiatrist and psychotherapist who practices in Würzburg, Germany, has studied parental alienation in Germany.

J. Michael Bone, Ph.D., is a clinical and forensic consultant who practices in Winter Park, Florida. Dr. Bone has worked for the last two decades as an evaluator, expert witness, therapist, researcher, and teacher specializing in the problem of parental alienation.

Barry Bricklin, Ph.D., served on the faculties of Jefferson Medical College and Hospital, Hahnemann Medical College, and Widener University, and was a guest lecturer at Temple University and Johns Hopkins University. He is the author of dozens of books, book chapters, tests, and journal articles on child custody issues.

Tamara Brockhausen, Psy.D., is a clinical and forensic psychologist who works in São Paulo, Brazil. She earned her degree at the Pontifícia Universidade Católica de São Paulo. Dr. Brockhausen is currently studying and conducting research on psychoanalysis and parental alienation at the Universidade de São Paulo. Also, she has served as a mediator at the family law court in São Paulo.

Andrew J. Chambers, M.D., J.D., is an attorney who recently graduated from Vanderbilt University School of Medicine.

Arantxa Coca Vila, an educational psychologist who works in Barcelona, Spain, is certified in psychological investigation. She has co-authored two books regarding parental alienation.

Douglas Darnall, Ph.D., is a psychologist who practices in Youngstown, Ohio. He wrote *Divorce Casualties: Protecting Your Children from Parental Alienation* and other books on this topic.

Gagan Dhaliwal, M.D., is a child and adolescent psychiatrist and forensic psychiatrist who practices in Huntsville, Alabama. He is an assistant clinical professor at the University of Alabama School of Medicine.

Benoit van Dieren, Ph.D., a psychologist, is a family therapist, family mediator, and expert who practices in Brussels, Belgium. He has studied parental alienation in Canada and Belgium.

Christian T. Dum, Ph.D., studied psychology and physics at the University of Vienna and the Massachusetts Institute of Technology. He is a former professor of theoretical physics at Cornell University. He currently is the head of an organization in Germany that deals with the psychological and legal aspects of child custody.

John E. Dunne, M.D., a child and adolescent psychiatrist in private practice in Tukwila, Washington, is a clinical associate professor of psychiatry at the University of Washington. Dr. Dunne was one of the authors of the Washington State Parenting Act of 1987, which altered the method for assigning parenting responsibilities for children post-divorce.

Robert A. Evans, Ph.D., is a school psychologist and mental health counselor who practices in Palm Harbor and other sites in Florida. He has testified in several states regarding parental alienation syndrome and child custody issues. Dr. Evans is an approved provider for continuing education for psychologists through the American Psychological Association and has been approved by bar associations to provide continuing legal education regarding parental alienation and parental alienation syndrome.

Robert Bruce Fane, Ed.D., a counseling psychologist who practices in Bowling Green, Kentucky, conducts child custody evaluations and other forensic evaluations. He has conducted research regarding domestic violence and substance abuse.

Bradley W. Freeman, M.D., is a child and adolescent psychiatrist and forensic psychiatrist who practices in Nashville, Tennessee. He is an assistant professor in the Department of Psychiatry, Vanderbilt University School of Medicine.

Laurence L. Greenhill, M.D., a child and adolescent psychiatrist, is Professor of Clinical Psychiatry at Columbia University. He is also the director of the Research Unit of Pediatric Psychopharmacology at Columbia University and New York State Psychiatric Hospital. Currently, Dr. Greenhill is the president of the American Academy of Child and Adolescent Psychiatry.

Guglielmo Gulotta, Full Professor, is a psychologist, lawyer, psychotherapist, and professor of forensic psychology at the University of Turin, Italy.

Anja Hannuniemi, LL.Lic., is a lawyer, licentiate of law, and medical law researcher and teacher at the University of Helsinki. She has studied parental alienation in Finland and is preparing a doctor's thesis regarding that topic.

Lena Hellblom Sjögren, Ph.D., is an investigative forensic psychologist and a researcher who works independently in Sweden and occasionally in Norway and other countries. She has identified 60 cases involving PAS, which she is analyzing in a research project that focuses on the violation of the child's human rights when the child is alienated from a parent without just cause.

Lawrence Hellmann, J.D., a noted legal researcher regarding child custody issues, works in Vista, California. His research contributed to five cases before the Supreme Court of California and one before the Supreme Court of the United States. He has also served as president of the National Congress for Fathers and Children.

Steve Herman, Ph.D., is an assistant professor in the Department of Psychology at the University of Hawaii at Hilo. He has conducted research on the methodology of child sexual abuse evaluations.

Adolfo Jarne Esparcia, Ph.D., is a professor at the University of Barcelona. He has written extensively regarding the practice of clinical psychology, including the *Manual de Psicopatologia Clinica and Psicopatologia.*

Allan M. Josephson, M.D., is a professor and the director of Child, Adolescent and Family Psychiatry at the University of Louisville School of Medicine, Louisville, Kentucky. He has published in the areas of family therapy, adolescent psychopathology, and spirituality and psychiatry. Dr. Josephson previously was the co-chair of the Family Committee of the American Academy of Child and Adolescent Psychiatry.

Joseph Kenan, M.D., is a child and adolescent psychiatrist and forensic psychiatrist who practices in Beverly Hills, California. Dr. Kenan is president of the American Society for Adolescent Psychiatry.

Ursula Kodjoe, M.A., is a family therapist, mediator, and family court expert who works in Emmendingen/Freiburg, Germany. She has studied parental alienation in Germany.

Douglas A. Kramer, M.D., M.S., a child, adolescent, and family psychiatrist practicing in Madison, Wisconsin, is a clinical professor of psychiatry at the University of Wisconsin School of Medicine and Public Health. He has written extensively on family issues and family psychotherapy. Dr. Kramer is the co-chair of the Family Committee of the American Academy of Child and Adolescent Psychiatry.

Ken Lewis, Ph.D., the director of Child Custody Evaluations Services of Philadelphia, Inc., has been a full-time custody evaluator and guardian *ad litem* since 1978. He has qualified as an expert witness in this field in 26 states and Canada. Dr. Lewis has authored books, book chapters, and journal articles on child custody issues, and has been a guest expert on several Webinars during International Parental Alienation Awareness Day.

Moira Liberatore, Psy.D., is a psychologist, psychotherapist, mediator, trial consultant, and lecturer at the University of Turin, Italy.

Demosthenes Lorandos, Ph.D., J.D., is a psychologist and attorney who works in Ann Arbor, Michigan. Dr. Lorandos has been a clinical and forensic psychologist for four decades. As an attorney, he is licensed in New York, California, and Michigan as well as a member of the bar of the United States Supreme Court.

Ludwig F. Lowenstein, Ph.D., a clinical psychologist who works in Eastleigh, Hampshire, United Kingdom, has studied parental alienation in the United Kingdom.

Domènec Luengo Ballester, Ph.D., a psychologist who works in Barcelona, Spain, has a particular interest in the treatment of anxiety disorders. Also, he has co-authored two books regarding parental alienation.

James C. MacIntyre, II, M.D., is a child and adolescent psychiatrist who practices in Charlotte, North Carolina. He is the secretary of the American Academy of Child and Adolescent Psychiatry.

Jayne A. Major, Ph.D., a consultant and educator who practices in Los Angeles, California, is the founder of Breakthrough Parenting Services and Stop Parental Alienation of Children. She is the author of numerous articles on parental alienation and parental alienation syndrome.

Eric G. Mart, Ph.D., is a forensic psychologist in private practice in Manchester, New Hampshire. Child custody assessment is a major part of his practice and he is the author of *Issue Focused Forensic Child Custody Assessment.*

Kim Masters, M.D., a child and adolescent psychiatrist, is the medical director of Three Rivers Midlands Campus Residential Treatment Center. Dr. Masters is an adjunct assistant clinical professor at the Physician Assistant Program, Medical College of South Carolina.

David McMillan, Ph.D., is a clinical psychologist who works in Nashville, Tennessee.

John E. Meeks, M.D., is a child and adolescent psychiatrist who practices in Rockville, Maryland. He has published books regarding psychotherapy with adolescents, depression in adolescents, the education of youngsters with emotional problems, and understanding adopted teenagers. Dr. Meeks is the founder and senior medical advisor of The Foundation Schools, Rockville, Maryland.

Steven G. Miller, M.D., is an internist and medical educator. He has 30 years of experience in forensic medicine, and for 15 years directed a consulting group in forensic psychiatry and psychology. Dr. Miller, who is board certified in internal medicine and emergency medicine, is a Clinical Instructor of Medicine at Harvard Medical School, Boston, Massachusetts.

Martha J. Morelock, Ph.D., works in the Department of Psychiatry, Vanderbilt University School of Medicine. Dr. Morelock's doctoral degree is in child development, specializing in cognitive and social-emotional development in children.

Stephen L. Morrison, Ph.D., is a supervisory sergeant with the Robbery Division of the Houston, Texas, Police Department. His doctoral degree is in the Administration of Justice, and Dr. Morrison is on the adjunct faculty of the Criminal Justice and Social Science Departments at the University of Houston - Downtown. He has conducted research regarding parental alienation.

Wade Myers, M.D., is a child and adolescent psychiatrist and forensic psychiatrist who practices in Providence, Rhode Island. He is a professor in the Department of Psychiatry at the Warren Alpert Medical School of Brown University.

Olga Odinetz, Ph.D., is a research scientist in health and environment who works in the *Institut de Recherche pour le Développement* in Paris, France. She is the founding president of the *Association Contre l'Aliénation Parentale* (ACALPA), a governmentally approved organization that engages in extensive education of parents, security officers, legal professionals, and mental health professionals regarding parental alienation.

Jeff Opperman, an author who works in Danbury, Connecticut, has published articles regarding parenting, divorce, parental alienation, and advocacy in *Counseling Today* and *The Richmond County Bar Association Journal.* His work has appeared on both *womansdivorce.com* and *dadsdivorce.com.* A former member of the board of directors of the Rachel Foundation, Mr. Opperman's personal story was featured on CNN and other media. He is a graduate student in counseling at Western Connecticut State University.

Judith M. Pilla, Ph.D., L.S.W., PMHCNS-BC, is a clinical social worker and clinical nurse specialist who practices in King of Prussia, Pennsylvania. Dr. Pilla has provided psychotherapy for individuals, couples, and families for 20 years. She leads couples groups regarding relationship issues, including parenting and communication in estranged relationships. She also consults with physicians, nurses, social service personnel, and medical agencies regarding communication problems between medical professionals and patients.

Robert L. Sain, M.D., is a child and adolescent psychiatrist who practices in Ann Arbor, Michigan. He is president and founder of Lifelines, Inc., a consultation service for programs and agencies that serve the state's most troubled children.

S. Richard Sauber, Ph.D., a Harvard trained, forensic psychologist, has a national practice. His office is in Boca Raton, Florida. He is the founding and current editor of *The American Journal of Family Therapy*. He was formerly a professor of psychiatry (psychology) at the Warren Alpert Medical School of Brown University, the Columbia University College of Physicians and Surgeons, and the University of Pennsylvania School of Medicine.

Thomas E. Schacht, Psy.D., is a clinical psychologist and forensic psychologist who practices in Johnson City, Tennessee. Dr. Schacht is a professor in the Department of Psychiatry and Behavioral Sciences at the James H. Quillen College of Medicine, East Tennessee State University.

Ulrich C. Schoettle, M.D., a child and adolescent psychiatrist who practices in Seattle, Washington, is a clinical professor in the Department of Psychiatry at the University of Washington. He has written on the topics of children of divorce and termination of parental rights.

Jesse Shaver, Ph.D., M.D., a research scientist in Nashville, Tennessee, is pursuing a career in ophthalmology.

Richard K. Stephens, a historian who lives in New York City, specializes in the history of family dismemberment, i.e., the removal of a child from a family context either by a relative or an unrelated agent. He is writing a book on the history of parental kidnapping and its cultural representations.

Julie Lounds Taylor, Ph.D., is an assistant professor in the Department of Pediatrics at Vanderbilt University School of Medicine. She is a statistical consultant for the Vanderbilt Kennedy Center.

Asunción Tejedor Huerta, Ph.D., a forensic psychologist who practices in Asturias, Spain, has studied parental alienation in Spain, Columbia, and Mexico. She has published books and articles in legal journals on this topic, and has taught courses for the Official College of Psychologists in Spain.

William M. Tucker, M.D., an ophthalmologist who practices in Syracuse, New York, is board certified in internal medicine and ophthalmology. He has taught residents, medical students, physicians' assistants, and nurse practitioners for over 20 years.

Hubert Van Gijseghem, Ph.D., is a forensic psychologist who was a professor at the University of Montreal. He has served as an expert in hundreds of legal cases involving parental alienation in Canada and Europe.

James S. Walker, Ph.D., is a forensic psychologist and neuropsychologist who practices in Nashville, Tennessee. He is an assistant professor in the Departments of Psychiatry, Psychology, and Neurology at Vanderbilt University School of Medicine.

Randy Warren, J.D., is a litigation attorney who practices law in San Rafael, California. He has dealt with child custody and parental alienation in his California court cases.

Monty N. Weinstein, Psy.D., FAPA, is a forensic expert who practices in New York and Georgia. He is a member of the editorial advisory board of the *Annals of the American Psychotherapy Association.* Dr. Weinstein has written extensively on terrorism and violence.

Jack C. Westman, M.D., is Professor Emeritus of Psychiatry at the University of Wisconsin School of Medicine and Public Health. He has published extensively on individual differences in children, learning disabilities, child abuse and neglect, child advocacy, family therapy, children's and parents' rights and public policy. He has been the editor of *Child Psychiatry and Human Development* and served as president of the American Association of Psychiatric Services for Children. Dr. Westman currently is president of Wisconsin Cares, Inc.

Katie Wilson, M.D., is a child and adolescent psychiatrist who practices in Nashville, Tennessee.

Robert H. Woody, Ph.D., Sc.D., J.D., is a professor in the Department of Psychology at the University of Nebraska at Omaha. He is also an attorney in private practice in Omaha, Nebraska.

Abe Worenklein, Ph.D., a clinical and forensic psychologist, is a professor in the Department of Psychology at Dawson College, Montreal, Canada, and an adjunct professor in the Department of Psychology at Concordia University, Montreal, Canada.

INTRODUCTION

Parental alienation is an important phenomenon that mental health professionals should know about and thoroughly understand, especially those who work with children, adolescents, divorced adults, and adults whose parents divorced when they were children. In this book, we define parental alienation as a mental condition in which a child—usually one whose parents are engaged in a high-conflict divorce—allies himself or herself strongly with one parent (the preferred parent) and rejects a relationship with the other parent (the alienated parent) without legitimate justification. This process leads to a tragic outcome when the child and the alienated parent, who previously had a loving and mutually satisfying relationship, lose the nurture and joy of that relationship for many years and perhaps for their lifetimes. We estimate that 1 percent of children and adolescents in the U.S. experience parental alienation. When the phenomenon is properly recognized, this condition is preventable and treatable in many instances.

There has been considerable discussion and debate regarding parental alienation among mental health and legal professionals. In order to understand the debate, it is important to know the difference between *parental alienation* and *parental alienation syndrome* as these terms are used in this book. The latter refers to a child with parental alienation who manifests several characteristic behaviors that have been said to constitute a syndrome. Also, the concept of parental alienation syndrome typically includes a causative factor, i.e., the alienating parent. This book discusses both parental alienation and parental alienation syndrome. While there has been almost universal acceptance of the reality and importance of parental alienation, there has been disagreement and debate regarding parental alienation syndrome. These discussions and debates have occurred for many years: parental alienation has been an issue in legal cases since at least the 1820s; parental alienation has been discussed in the mental health literature since the 1940s; parental alienation syndrome has been discussed and debated since the 1980s.

The authors of this book believe that parental alienation is not simply a minor aberration in the life of a family, but a serious mental condition. Because of the false belief that the alienated parent is a dangerous or unworthy person, the child loses one of the most important relationships in his or her life. The alienated parent is at risk for experiencing chronic depression and anxiety. There have been scores of research studies and hundreds of scholarly articles, chapters, and books regarding parental alienation and parental alienation syndrome. Although we have located professional publications from about thirty countries on six continents, we agree that research should continue regarding this important mental condition that affects hundreds of thousands of children and their families.

The time has come for the concepts of parental alienation and parental alienation syndrome to be included in the *Diagnostic and Statistical Manual of Mental Disorders,* Fifth Edition (DSM-5) and the *International Classification of Diseases,* Eleventh Edition (ICD-11). This book provides in detail the bases for this recommendation.

With regard to the *Diagnostic and Statistical Manual of Mental Disorders,* Fifth Edition (DSM-5), a group of mental health and legal professionals were invited to submit a formal proposal to the DSM-5 Disorders in Childhood and Adolescence Work Group. The proposal, "Parental Alienation Disorder and DSM-V," was submitted to the Work Group in August 2008. The August 2008 formal proposal included more than 50 citations and quotations from the mental health literature and more than 90 citations from the world legal literature. The authors concluded that the diversity of these publications supported the proposition that the concept of parental alienation is generally accepted by mental health and legal professionals. The August 2008 proposal was published in *The American Journal of Family Therapy* (Bernet, 2008).

After reviewing the August 2008 formal proposal, Daniel Pine, M.D., the chairman of the Disorders in Childhood and Adolescence Work Group, replied that the original proposal did not have enough information about the validity of parental alienation as a distinct mental condition, the reliability of the diagnostic criteria, and the prevalence of this condition. Dr. Pine provided constructive criticism to the authors of the proposal, and suggested that we either locate or conduct additional research regarding this topic. Dr. Pine indicated that the Work Group would be pleased to consider this additional research as they continue their deliberations regarding the child and adolescent aspects of DSM-5.

With regard to the *International Classification of Diseases,* Eleventh Edition (ICD-11) of the World Health Organization, we are aware that there is considerable interest in coordinating as much as possible the content of DSM-5 and ICD-11. With that in mind, the authors were invited to submit a proposal regarding parental alienation to the WHO International Advisory Group for the Revision of ICD-10 Mental and Behavioural Disorders. This document–*Parental Alienation, DSM-5, and ICD-11*–has been submitted both to the DSM-5 Task Force and the ICD-11 International Advisory Group.

This book is based on the August 2008 proposal, "Parental Alienation Disorder and DSM-V," but is longer and much more detailed. This document contains much more information about the validity, reliability, and prevalence of parental alienation. It also includes a comprehensive international bibliography regarding parental alienation with more than 600 citations. Part of this document was published in *The American Journal of Family Therapy* (Bernet et al., 2010). In order to bring life to the definitions and the technical writing, this book also contains several short clinical vignettes. These vignettes are based on actual families and real events, but have been modified to protect the privacy of both the parents and children. In some instances, two or more cases have been merged into a single vignette.

ACKNOWLEDGMENTS

This project began in June 2008, shortly after the American Psychiatric Association announced the membership of the various work groups that constitute the DSM-5 Task Force. Since then, a large number of colleagues have contributed to the two previous publications regarding parental alienation, DSM-5, and ICD-11 (Bernet, 2008; Bernet et al., 2010) and to this book, which is the most detailed publication to date addressing this topic.

When I was considering writing a proposal that parental alienation be included in DSM-5, I contacted two of the editors of *The International Handbook of Parental Alienation,* Demosthenes Lorandos and S. Richard Sauber. They encouraged me to forge ahead with this project and provided invaluable advice and guidance as we developed the formal proposals, the journal publications, and this book.

During these two years, the most important single event was an informal gathering that occurred in Florence, Italy, in April 2009. Wilfrid von Boch-Galhau, a psychiatrist from Germany, arranged a meeting of colleagues from several European countries. This international colloquium regarding parental alienation included: Eduard Bakalář (Czech Republic), Paul Bensussan (France), Benoit van Dieren (Belgium), Christian Dum (Germany), Anja Hannuniemi (Finland), Lena Hellblom Sjögren (Sweden), Ursula Kodjoe (Germany), and Olga Odinetz (France). In that meeting, it was obvious that mental health and legal professionals from many countries had observed the exact same phenomenon—that is, children of parents engaged in a high-conflict divorce may become alienated from a loving parent and lose their relationship with that parent. By the end of the meeting in Florence, our group had agreed: to stay in touch; to enlarge the scope of our proposal to include international professional literature regarding parental alienation; and to address our proposal to both DSM-5 and ICD-11.

In subsequent months, my new friends in Europe contributed much of the content of this book, that is, legal and mental health publications regarding parental alienation from their respective countries. The "Committee of Florence" put me in touch with colleagues in Spain, Italy, the United

Kingdom, and Canada. I quickly learned that there is a robust international literature regarding parental alienation that U.S. mental health professionals know almost nothing about. As a group, we ultimately collected references from the professional literature of 30 countries from six continents. Christian Dum, in particular, helped me develop the bibliography for this book. Some of these scholars and practitioners–for example, Ludwig Lowenstein (United Kingdom), Guglielmo Gulotta (Italy), José M. Aguilar (Spain), and Abe Worenklein (Canada)–provided frequent, friendly encouragement.

There were many individuals in the U.S. who contributed their expertise to this project. Amy J. L. Baker provided information regarding adult children of parental alienation. Barry Bricklin sent me information about his own research. Douglas Darnall offered suggestions, advice, and encouragement. Ken Lewis tracked down hard-to-locate documents at the Library of Congress. Stephen L. Morrison helped to organize the research regarding the validity and reliability of the concepts of parental alienation and PAS. Richard K. Stephens provided fascinating historical legal records. Larry Hellman, Randy Warren, and Thomas E. Schacht wrote the section on legal aspects of parental alienation. Fifteen contributors provided short clinical and legal vignettes that have been included in this book. In a few instances, contributors described their personal experiences with parental alienation.

As clinicians and forensic experts, my colleagues who are child and adolescent psychiatrists have had much experience with patients and evaluees who manifested parental alienation. I sincerely appreciate the support I received from Douglas A. Kramer (co-author of the earliest description of parental alienation in a peer reviewed journal); John E. Dunne (co-author of early research on the treatment of parental alienation); E. James Anthony (who described *folie à deux,* which can cause severe parental alienation); Allan M. Josephson (an authority regarding family therapy); John E. Meeks (an authority in evaluating and treating adolescents); and Wade Myers (an authority in child and adolescent forensic psychiatry).

My colleagues at Vanderbilt University School of Medicine have been very helpful, particularly Stephan Heckers (chair of the Department of Psychiatry and an expert in psychiatric nosology); James S. Walker (a forensic psychologist), Bradley W. Freeman (a forensic child and adolescent psychiatrist), Martha J. Morelock (a psychologist who specialized in child development), and Julie Lounds Taylor (a statistics consultant). Several medical students and psychiatry trainees contributed to this project: Katie Wilson collected material for the bibliography; Jesse Shaver located important research regarding parental alienation; and Andrew J. Chambers, both a lawyer and a medical student, developed Appendix C of this book, the summaries of legal cases. John Howser and Craig Boerner facilitated our interaction with the media. My assistant, Allison Kee, helped me in many ways to stay focused on this project and to cope with a myriad of administrative details.

Finally, my family has been supportive. My wife, Susan Bernet (a psychiatric nurse), and daughter, Alice C. Bernet (a graduate student at Vanderbilt University School of Nursing), helped me develop the extensive bibliography regarding parental alienation. My daughter-in-law, Kristin C. Bernet (a librarian with Johns Hopkins University), tracked down obscure citations, even when the authors of the articles were unable to provide the information.

This book was a group effort of a large number of colleagues and collaborators in addition to the individuals mentioned here. I thank you all for your patience and perseverance in contributing to this important project.

WILLIAM BERNET, M.D.
Nashville, Tennessee

PARENTAL ALIENATION, DSM-5, AND ICD-11

Chapter One

DEFINITIONS AND GOALS

Although parental alienation has been described in the psychiatric literature for at least 60 years, it has never been considered for inclusion in the *Diagnostic and Statistical Manual of Mental Disorders* (DSM). When DSM-IV was being developed, nobody formally proposed that parental alienation be included in that edition. Since the publication of DSM-IV in 1994, there have been hundreds of publications (articles, chapters, books, court opinions) regarding parental alienation in peer reviewed mental health journals, legal literature, and the popular press. There has been controversy among mental health and legal professionals regarding some aspects of parental alienation, and at times the professional discourse resembled the hostility manifested by entrenched and angry parents fighting over their children.

Regarding our proposed diagnostic criteria, we say that the essential feature of *parental alienation* is that a child—usually one whose parents are engaged in a high-conflict divorce—allies himself or herself strongly with one parent (the preferred parent) and rejects a relationship with the other parent (the alienated parent) without legitimate justification. The primary behavioral symptom is that the child refuses or resists contact with a parent, or has contact with a parent that is characterized either by extreme withdrawal or gross contempt. The primary mental symptom is the child's irrational anxiety and/or hostility toward the rejected parent. This anxiety and hostility may have been brought about by the preferred parent or by other circumstances, such as the child who avoids being caught between warring parents by gravitating to one side and avoiding the other side of the conflict.

In this document, we differentiate the general concept of *parental alienation* and *parental alienation syndrome*. Parental alienation refers to the child's strong alliance with one parent and rejection of a relation-ship with the other parent without legitimate justification. Depending on the context, we sometimes use the term *parental alienation syndrome* (PAS), which is a more complex concept. When we refer to the research and published literature, we use the term PAS if that was the terminology in the original material.

PAS typically refers to a child with parental alienation who mani-fests some or all of eight characteristic behaviors, which include: the child's campaign of denigration against the alienated parent; frivolous rationalizations for the child's criticism of the alienated parent; lack of ambivalence; the independent-thinker phenomenon; reflexive sup-port of the preferred parent against the alienated parent; an absence of guilt over exploitation and mistreatment of the alienated parent; bor-rowed scenarios; and spread of the child's animosity toward the alien-ated parent's extended family (Gardner, 1992a). (These eight behav-iors or symptoms are defined in Appendix A of this book.) Another difference between parental alienation and PAS is that the latter typi-cally includes the idea that one of the parents actively influenced the child to fear and avoid the other parent. Although we believe that occurs in many instances, it is not necessary to have an alienating par-ent for parental alienation to occur. Parental alienation may occur sim-ply in the context of a high-conflict divorce in which the parents fight and the child aligns with one side to get out of the middle of the bat-tle, even with no indoctrination by the favored parent.

Parental alienation and PAS do not describe or pertain to different groups of children. On the contrary, we believe that the children who experience parental alienation are almost exactly the same children who manifest PAS. The latter is a subset of the former. We believe that the great majority of children who experience parental alienation also manifest some or all of the eight characteristic behaviors of PAS. In other words, parental alienation is simply a general term that is not encumbered by the baggage associated with PAS, i.e., the eight symp-toms that constitute the syndrome and the role of the alienating par-ent. In our use of these terms, parental alienation and PAS are typi-cally descriptors of the child. (For example, "For several years, Jimmy lost the loving relationship he had with his mother because of parental alienation.") However, the terms could be used to describe the triadic relationship that involves two parents and a child. (For example, "Every member of the Smith family was damaged by a severe degree of parental alienation.")

We are explaining these definitions in detail because we realize that some authors have given other meanings to "parental alienation." For example, some authors use "parental alienation" to describe the behaviors of the alienating parent and "PAS" to describe the condition of the child. Also, some authors use "parental alienation" to describe any estrangement between the child and a parent (including situations in which the parent was abusive) and "PAS" to describe the child's unjustified rejection of a parent (i.e., when the parent was not abusive).

When we refer to our proposal for DSM-5 and ICD-11, we use the term *parental alienation disorder* (because that is the terminology for mental disorders in DSM-5) or *parental alienation relational problem* (because that is the terminology for relational problems in DSM-5). See Appendix A for the proposed criteria for parental alienation disorder. See Appendix B for the proposed criteria for parental alienation relational problem. The proposed criteria for parental alienation disorder and parental alienation relational problem are partly based on the definition of PAS.

We use the phrase *contact refusal* for the behavior of the child or adolescent who adamantly avoids spending time with one of the parents. Contact refusal is simply a symptom that could have a number of possible causes, one of which is parental alienation. This terminology is similar to *school refusal,* which is simply a symptom that could have a number of possible causes.

In February 2010, the American Psychiatric Association changed the abbreviation for the next edition of DSM. It had previously been referred to as "DSM-V," but the organization changed the abbreviation to "DSM-5" when the new website, *www.dsm5.org,* was introduced. In this book, we use "DSM-V" when that was the term in the original source material, such as the name of a publication or a quotation. We use "DSM-5" when referring to the future, i.e., the next edition of DSM.

Our proposal is that one of the following will occur with regard to DSM-5:

- The text in Appendix A (regarding parental alienation disorder) will be included in the main body of DSM-5.
- OR, the text in Appendix A will be included in one of the appendices of DSM-5, that is, Criteria Sets and Axes for Further Study.

- OR, the text in Appendix B (regarding parental alienation relational problem) will be included in the chapter of DSM-5, Other Conditions That May Be a Focus of Clinical Attention.

The DSM-V website (*www.psych.org/MainMenu/Research/DSMIV/DSMV.aspx*) includes a document, "Guidelines for Making Changes to DSM-V" (Kendler at al., 2009), which discusses the criteria that DSM-5 personnel should consider in adopting a new diagnosis. In Chapter Three of this book, we list these criteria and explain how they are fulfilled by parental alienation.

In addition to being included in DSM-5 as either a mental disorder or a relational problem, the concept of parental alienation should be mentioned in the DSM-5 differential diagnoses of certain disorders seen in children and adolescents. For instance, parental alienation should be mentioned in the differential diagnosis of separation anxiety disorder, since both conditions can be manifested by an apparent fear of leaving one of the parents. Parental alienation should be mentioned in the differential diagnosis of oppositional defiant disorder, since both conditions can be manifested by the child's adamant refusal to follow a reasonable expectation of an adult.

We are making an analogous proposal regarding ICD-11:

- The text in Appendix A (regarding parental alienation disorder) will be included in the section of Chapter V called "Behavioural and emotional disorders with onset usually occurring in childhood and adolescence."
- OR, the text in Appendix B (regarding parental alienation relational problem) will be included in one of the sections of Chapter XXI. For example, Chapter XXI includes a section called "Other problems related to primary support group, including family circumstances" and another section called "Problems related to other legal circumstances." Parental alienation relational problem would be appropriate for one of those sections.

We believe there is almost uniform consensus in the international mental health community that parental alienation is a real phenomenon that affects the life-long mental health of thousands of children and likewise the mental health of their families. Parental alienation affects the quality of life of those who are exposed to it. We believe there is enough research regarding validity, reliability, and prevalence to support the adoption of parental alienation as a psychiatric diagnosis.

Chapter Two

TWENTY REASONS WHY PARENTAL ALIENATION SHOULD BE A DIAGNOSIS

It is time to include parental alienation as a diagnosis in DSM-5 and ICD-11 for the following reasons:

1. Developmental factors are being considered for DSM-5. Attachment is a very important developmental factor, and parental alienation can be conceptualized as a disorder of attachment.

2. Relational problems are being considered for DSM-5, and parental alienation is a typical example of this type of mental condition.

3. Dimensional diagnoses are being considered for DSM-5, and the descriptions of parental alienation have had dimensional features since the early 1990s.

4. The phenomenon of parental alienation was described long before PAS was formally defined.

5. Parental alienation is a valid concept. There has been considerable qualitative and quantitative research regarding parental alienation and PAS.

6. Parental alienation is a valid concept. In the 1980s and 1990s, the phenomenon was recognized and described independently by at least six researchers or groups of researchers.

7. Parental alienation is a valid concept. After PAS was formally defined, many researchers or groups of researchers were able to apply the definition to their own subjects.

8. Parental alienation is a valid concept. Despite controversies

regarding terminology and etiology, the phenomenon is almost universally accepted by mental health professionals who evaluate and treat children of high-conflict divorces.

9. Parental alienation is a valid concept. Parental alienation has been identified and studied in many countries.

10. Parental alienation is a valid concept. Collateral research regarding related topics supports the contention that parental alienation is a real phenomenon.

11. The diagnostic criteria for PAS are reliable. Systematic research indicates the diagnostic criteria exhibit both test-retest and inter-rater reliability.

12. It is possible to estimate the prevalence of parental alienation. Systematic research indicates the prevalence of parental alienation in the U.S. is approximately 1% of children and adolescents.

13. Parental alienation and PAS have been discussed by professional organizations.

14. Parental alienation and PAS have been discussed extensively by legal professionals.

15. Parental alienation and PAS have been discussed extensively by the general public.

16. Parental alienation is a serious mental condition. It has a predictable course that often continues into adulthood and can cause serious, long-term psychological problems.

17. Establishing diagnostic criteria will make it possible to study parental alienation in a systematic manner on a larger scale.

18. Establishing diagnostic criteria will be helpful for: clinicians who work with divorced families; divorced parents, who are trying to do what is best for their children; and children of divorce, who desperately need appropriate treatment that is based on a correct diagnosis.

19. Establishing diagnostic criteria should reduce the opportunities for abusive parents and unethical attorneys to misuse the concept of parental alienation in child custody disputes.

20. There are critics of parental alienation and PAS who oppose the use of these concepts as a psychiatric diagnosis, but their arguments are not convincing.

1. Developmental factors are being considered for DSM-5. Attachment is a very important developmental factor, and parental alienation can be conceptualized as a disorder of attachment.

Child and adolescent psychiatrists and other mental health professionals have urged DSM-5 personnel to take a developmental approach with regard to the diagnoses that apply to children and adolescents and the criteria for these diagnoses. For example, the criteria for some disorders are different, depending on whether the patient is a child or an adult.

One of the most important aspects of child and adolescent development is the concept of attachment, that is, the affective tie between a child and a caregiver. There are several psychiatric conditions that directly affect the child's attachment to caregivers or reflect an aberration in the child's attachment. The most obvious disorders of attachment are reactive attachment disorder (markedly disturbed and developmentally inappropriate social relatedness in most contexts) and separation anxiety disorder (excessive anxiety concerning separation from . . . those to whom the individual is attached). There are other disorders that may be considered disorders of attachment, such as feeding disorder of infancy or early childhood (because the condition may be caused by parent-child interaction problems) and oppositional defiant disorder (because the condition may be caused by harsh, inconsistent, or neglectful child-rearing practices).

We recommend that, in DSM-5, attachment disorders be clustered in the same way that pervasive developmental disorders and elimination disorders are clustered in DSM-IV-TR. This new section would start with a general overview of the significance of attachment as a developmental issue, a brief discussion of typical attachment phenomena in childhood and adolescence, and a general explanation of the problematic variations in attachment. Parental alienation disorder can be conceptualized as a disorder of attachment and included in this cluster of mental disorders. It is notable that all of these disorders of attachment have something important in common, that is, they are not predominantly genetic or constitutional, but are caused primarily by what parents or caretakers do and say to their children.

2. Relational problems are being considered for DSM-5. Parental alienation is a typical example of a relational problem because it usually involves the interacting attitudes of one child and two parents.

In DSM-IV-TR, relational problems were included as V codes in the chapter, Other Conditions That May Be a Focus of Clinical Attention. For example, one of the relational problems in DSM-IV-TR is parent-child relational problem (V61.20). According to DSM-IV-TR, "This category should be used when the focus of clinical attention is a pattern of interaction between parent and child . . . that is associated with clinically significant impairment in individual or family functioning or the development of clinically significant symptoms in parent or child" (American Psychiatric Association, 2000, page 737).

It is our understanding that relational problems will be addressed in a more comprehensive manner in DSM-5. One way to organize DSM-5 would be to have a separate chapter called Relational Problems. That chapter could explain the difference between mental disorders and relational problems, and also explain how relational factors are a consideration in many mental disorders.

Recent publications by DSM-5 personnel emphasized the importance of relational problems. For example, Michael First and his colleagues said, "Relational disorders are painful, persistent behavioral problems that seriously affect adjustment and should be considered for inclusion in the next edition of the DSM" (First et al., 2002). Also, we agree with Steven Beach and his colleagues that "disorder-specific relationship processes may prove to be critical for understanding particular disorders or for distinguishing functionally distinct types of disorders. Accordingly, a . . . proposal for enhancing the description of relationship processes in DSM-V would incorporate a reference to the presence or absence of disorder-specific relational processes with relational specifiers" (Beach et al., 2006). Beach et al. gave examples of diagnoses–feeding disorder of infancy and conduct disorder–that have prominent relational characteristics.

In considering how relational problems will be presented in DSM-5, parental alienation should be at the forefront of the discussion. Parental alienation can be conceptualized simply as a mental disorder of the child, who has a false belief that one of his or her parents is a dangerous or contemptible or simply expendable person. Or, parental alienation can be conceptualized as a complex relational problem in which: two parents have a highly conflicted relationship; the child has a pathologically enmeshed relationship with the preferred parent; and the child has an unfounded fear or disregard of the alienated parent. Furthermore, all three parties contribute in some way to the end result of the child's false belief.

It is not a new idea that the concept of parent-child relational problem (V61.20) overlaps to some extent with the concept of parental alienation. Richard Gardner commented on this topic in his article, "Does DSM-IV have equivalents for the parental alienation syndrome (PAS) diagnosis?" Gardner thought that parent-child relational problem and PAS "have some symptoms in common," but they are not equivalent. He said, "In the PAS situation there is a pathological dyad between the alienating parent and the child and another pathological dyad between the alienated parent and the child. . . . Examiners using this criterion do well to emphasize that two separate parent-child relational problems are manifested" (Gardner, 2003a).

The Comprehensive Textbook of Psychiatry suggests that parent-child relational problem includes the symptoms and behaviors that are typically seen in parental alienation. In the chapter on Relational Problems, the author said, "Substantial evidence indicates that marital discord leads to problems in children, from depression and withdrawal to conduct disorder and poor performance at school. This negative effect may be partly mediated through *triangulation* of the parent-child relationships. *Triangulation* refers to the process in which conflicted parents attempt to win the sympathy and support of their child, who is recruited by one parent as an ally in the struggle with the partner" (Dickstein, 2005, page 2244). At least one medical insurance company specifically states in its provider handbook that PAS is an example of parent-child relational problem. The *ValueOptions Provider Handbook* states the following example in the section regarding parent-child relational problem: "Unresolved parental conflict (i.e., the constant devaluing of one parent by the other) in divorced or estranged families resulting in parental alienation syndrome" (ValueOptions, 2006).

ICD already includes several conditions that are comparable to the relational problems in DSM-IV. Chapter XXI of ICD-10 includes a section called "Problems related to negative life events in childhood," which includes "Altered pattern of family relationships in childhood"

(Z61.2). There is a section called "Other problems related to primary support group, including family circumstances," which includes "Disruption of family by separation or divorce" (Z63.5). In fact, disruption of family by separation or divorce has an explanatory note that refers to "estrangement." It is unclear what "estrangement" means in this context and whether the authors of ICD-10 have already included the concept of parental alienation in their understanding of disruption of family by separation or divorce. Finally, there is a section called "Problems related to other psychosocial circumstances," which includes "Problems related to other legal circumstances" (Z65.3). The last category, problems related to other legal circumstances, makes reference to "child custody or support proceedings."

Although both DSM and ICD allude to relational problems and although parental alienation is a classic example of severe relational

---

Father Alienates Children from Mother
Monty N. Weinstein, Psy.D., Brooklyn, New York

Dr. Weinstein was asked to consult regarding a post-divorce case in Wyoming. The mother had no parenting time because the father claimed the children did not want to see her. Dr. Weinstein extensively interviewed the children in Wyoming. When he testified regarding this case, Dr. Weinstein explained how the father had programmed the children against their mother. According to Dr. Weinstein, the father portrayed the mother—using subliminal suggestions—as a diabolical creature. The court accepted this analysis and ordered that the mother have reasonable parenting time with the children.

Here are some examples of "subliminal suggestions": "Your Mom's not much fun, is she?" "Your Mom didn't call you today, did she?" "Your Mom didn't take you to the doctor when you had a cough, did she?" "We had a great time at the zoo today, didn't we? Your Mom wasn't with us, though, was she?"

This case reminds us that parental indoctrination can be subtle and may begin before the physical separation of the parents. A tone of voice, a disparaging look, or an offhand comment can all contribute to alienating a child from the targeted parent. The indoctrination process can be both a conscious effort and an unconscious occurrence.

---

problems, neither DSM nor ICD explicitly mentions parental alienation. We recommend that the committees charged with coordinating DSM-5 and ICD-11 find a way to include parental alienation in both of these documents.

3. **Dimensional diagnoses are being considered for DSM-5, and the descriptions of parental alienation have had dimensional features since the early 1990s.**

There has been discussion and debate for years as to whether psychiatric diagnoses should be organized following a categorical model or a dimensional model–or both. Helena Kraemer and colleagues explained, "A *categorical* approach to a diagnosis results in labeling each subject as either having (D+) or not having (D-) a disorder. . . . The DSM-IV categorizes a patient as being depressed or not depressed. A *dimensional* approach results in labeling each subject with an ordinal score (D), with high scores a stronger indicator of the presence of the disorder. Higher scores on the Hamilton depression scale are associated with a stronger likelihood of 'being depressed'" (Kraemer et al., 2004).

DSM-IV-TR already has some dimensional features, for example, in the current state of major depressive disorder (mild, moderate, severe without psychotic features, and severe with psychotic features) and in the severity of mental retardation (mild, moderate, severe, and profound). The various committees that are developing DSM-5 are apparently planning on adding additional dimensional aspects to our diagnostic system. In an important article, "A Dimensional Approach to Developmental Psychopathology," Hudziak et al. (2007) said, "We propose adding dimensional features to complement the categorical aspects of DSM. The dimensional and categorical approaches each have advantages and disadvantages. . . . We argue that a purely categorical approach fails to account for important sources of variance."

In keeping with this trend, various authors have described parental alienation in both categorical and dimensional terms since the early 1990s. In his book, *The Parental Alienation Syndrome,* Richard Gardner described three types of PAS, severe cases, moderate cases, and mild cases (Gardner, 1992a, pages 149–154). In their "reformulation" of parental alienation, Joan Kelly and Janet Johnston emphasized the continuum of parent-child relationships, with positive relationships at

Children Killed in Context of Custody Dispute
Stephen L. Morrison, Ph.D., Houston, Texas

In December 2009, there were multiple news reports that a woman, her two young daughters, and her mother were all found shot to death in their upscale home in San Clemente, California. In the initial investigation, it was not clear whether the children were killed by their mother or their maternal grandmother.

Earlier in the day, a court commissioner had tentatively ordered the mother, Ms. Elizabeth Fontaine, to relinquish temporary custody of her two young children to her ex-husband's sister. Ms. Fontaine was ordered to return to court with her daughters later in the day for a final ruling. The commissioner granted temporary custody of the girls to the paternal aunt, but—in the meantime—they were killed.

The girls' parents had engaged in a high-conflict custody dispute in which the mother repeatedly accused the father of molesting the two girls. During a trial, a court psychologist testified that molestation had not occurred and the court awarded primary custody to the mother, but allowed the father unmonitored visitation with the girls. The mother, however, had the children examined by new psychologists and renewed her allegations of molestation. Although the mother's allegations were taken seriously and investigated, no molestation charges were ever filed against the father.

This case is an extreme example, but it illustrates how parents may become intensely angry and determined when they fight over their children and through their children. Of course, the children become the victims when parents fight with each other.

one end and alienated relationships at the other (Kelly and Johnston, 2001). Although Gardner and Kelly and Johnston had different ways of conceptualizing parental alienation, they all highlighted the dimensional features of the phenomenon. With this in mind, it is clear that parental alienation fits into how DSM-5 is likely to be organized.

4. The phenomenon of parental alienation was described long before parental alienation syndrome was formally defined.

The phenomenon of parental alienation was described long before Richard Gardner coined the term "parental alienation syndrome" (Gardner, 1985). The features of parental alienation were described in legal cases 200 years ago. The phenomenon of parental alienation has been noted in the mental health literature for at least 60 years.

Historical Legal Cases

Richard K. Stephens, a historian in New York City, has studied records related to family conflict and parental kidnapping from the eighteenth century to the present time. He found that in the nineteenth century, legal writers and journalists used various terms to refer to the phenomenon that we call parental alienation (Stephens, 2009a, 2009b). These fascinating historical vignettes from contemporaneous newspapers indicate that the concept of parental alienation has been understood by the general public for hundreds of years.

In an 1827 case in Canterbury, England, the parents of Emily Ball were divorced. Emily's mother reported "an illicit connexion between her husband and his niece"; Emily's father, in response, declared that the mother "had endeavoured to alienate the affections of the child from him" (*The Times,* London, England, August 7, 1827).

In an 1877 case in New York City, Mrs. Annette Guillot sued Mr. Modeste Guillot for divorce, alleging that he treated her cruelly. She charged her husband with "vilifying her character and poisoning the minds of their children against her" (*The New York Times,* October 16, 1877).

In an 1883 case in Brooklyn, New York, Mrs. Hyland and Mr. Charles Hyland were separated because of the "husband's brutal treatment." Mrs. Hyland alleged that Mr. Hyland "secreted the children for the purpose of alienating their affections from her" (*The Brooklyn Daily Eagle,* August 29, 1883).

A 1904 case was litigated in Tennessee, "Dakota," and ultimately New York. Mrs. Pauline Carter sued Mr. Arthur Carter for divorce and she sought custody of their 9-year-old son. Mrs. Carter alleged that Mr. Carter "has stolen the child and prejudiced him against her." The writer noted, "To illustrate how Carter had poisoned her child's mind against her, she told of one instance when the boy threatened to shoot her, and was only prevented by some one standing near." Also, that Mr. Carter "and his family have exercised an undue influence over the boy and has inoculated [him] with hatred toward her, so that he is now not desirous of seeing her" (*New York Tribune,* July 29, 1904).

Case of Parental Alienation Prompts
Child Custody Law Reform
Richard Stephens, New York, New York

An important historical case pertaining to parental alienation was *Westmeath v. Westmeath* (1818), which involved British aristocracy. The parents were George Nugent, Marquess of Westmeath, and Emily Cecil, daughter of the Marquess of Salisbury. They married in 1812 and their daughter, Rosa, was born in 1814. It was reported that George physically assaulted Emily and committed adultery. Although they did not divorce, they separated in 1818 with the agreement that Emily would be the custodial parent of Rosa. However, George became convinced that Emily was poisoning Rosa's mind against him, so he refused to return the child to the mother after a visitation. Emily immediately sought a writ of habeas corpus, but the judge overrode the standing written agreement and awarded custody to the father. In that era, fathers typically had custody of children following divorce and the judge adopted the position that fathers cannot contract away their paternal rights. Also, George accused Emily of having an affair with the Duke of Wellington, which was apparently a false allegation.

Based on the legal records and other documents regarding this famous case, we can say that Rosa developed severe parental alienation. George isolated Rosa from her mother by moving her to the country home of his friend, the Duke of Buckingham. George instructed all in the household to never allow the mother, Emily, to see or communicate with the child. He apparently succeeded in thoroughly poisoning the child's mind against the mother. On two occasions, however, Emily forced her way into Rosa's new home. Rosa, about age 11, refused to kiss her mother or shake her hand. Emily later wrote that Rosa said to her, "Papa and the Duke of Buckingham have pointed out what sort of woman you were. I never wish to see your face again."

This case was associated with an important reform in British child custody law. Marchioness Emily Westmeath was a friend of Caroline Norton, a professional writer famous for her wit and beauty, who initiated and promoted the Infant Custody Bill, which was passed in 1839. The Infant Custody Bill—an important initiative that increased the rights of mothers regarding child custody—allowed mothers to appeal for custody of children under age 7 and access to children under age 16. Emily Westmeath took an active role in encouraging Parliament to pass the Infant Custody Bill. A summary of the Westmeath case with the description of "poisoning of the mind" can be found in *Broken Lives: Separation and Divorce in England, 1660–1857,* by Lawrence Stone (1993).

Wilhelm Reich, M.D.

In 1945, Wilhelm Reich, M.D., wrote in his classic book, *Charakteranalyse (Character Analysis)* (German), that some divorced parents defend themselves against narcissistic injury by fighting for custody of their child and defaming their former spouse. Although Reich had never heard of parental alienation, he described the phenomenon based on adults he had evaluated. In a chapter titled "Emotional Plague," Reich described both mothers and fathers who alienated their children against the other parent. Reich said, "Rescuing the child is regularly just a pretext and unfulfilled motive, as the result shows. The true motive is revenge on the partner through robbing him or her of the pleasure in the child. The fight over the child uses therefore the defamation of the partner, regardless whether he/she is healthy or sick. The lack of consideration for the child expresses itself in that his or her love for the other parent is not taken into account. The child is told, in order to alienate him or her from the partner, that this person is an alcoholic or psychotic, which does not correspond to the truth. The result is harm to the child, the motive is revenge on the partner and his/her destruction as well as control over the child, and not love for the child" (Reich, 1945, page 349).

Louise Despert, M.D.

In 1953, Louise Despert, M.D., referred in her book, *Children of Divorce,* to some aspects of parental alienation. She said, "It is a sharp temptation for the parent who remains with the child to break down their love for the one who has gone. As we have said several times before, this may be a temporary relief to the parent who does so, but it can do only harm to the child. It only keeps alive the bitterness and misunderstanding which cause parents and children so much pain in divorce" (Despert, 1953, page 52). Despert was a pioneer child psychiatrist who wrote extensively about childhood schizophrenia, psychotherapy with children, and children's reactions to the events of World War II.

Jack C. Westman, M.D., and Colleagues

Perhaps the first description of parental alienation in a peer-reviewed journal was an article by Jack C. Westman, M.D., David W.

Cline, M.D., William J. Swift, M.D., and Douglas A. Kramer, M.D., that was published in *The Archives of General Psychiatry,* "Role of Child Psychiatry in Divorce." These authors said, "Another pattern is found in which one parent and a child team up to produce an effect on the other parent. Not infrequently a child sides with one parent or the other, though feeling ambivalent underneath. In these cases one parent appears to deliberately undermine the other through a child" (Westman et al., 1970).

David J. Sheffner, M.D., and John M. Suarez, M.D.

Another early description of parental alienation in a peer-reviewed journal was a "brief communication" by David J. Sheffner and John M. Suarez, that was published in *The American Journal of Psychiatry,* "The Postdivorce Clinic." Sheffner and Suarez described a clinic that evaluated court-referred families who had child custody or visitation problems following divorce. The authors were affiliated with the University of California, Los Angeles, and they advised the domestic relations branch of the Los Angeles County Superior Court. One of the clinical vignettes in that article was a perfect example of parental alienation, although the authors, of course, did not call it that: "A woman who harbored much resentment toward her ex-husband influenced her young children against him. Both parents were well-functioning people and generally decent parents, except for the mother's irrational and destructive behavior in this one area. The children exprienced considerable anxiety when visiting their father and wanted to discontinue their relationship with him altogether. The father came to the domestic relations court for help" (Sheffner and Suarez, 1975).

E. Mavis Hetherington, Ph.D.

Since the early 1970s, E. Mavis Hetherington meticulously studied divorced parents and their children. Her research was called the Virginia Longitudinal Study of Divorce and Remarriage, which began in 1972, the Hetherington and Clingempeel Study of Divorce and Remarriage, and the Nonshared Environment Study. Although Hetherington did not use the term, "parental alienation," she noted and described some aspects of the phenomenon. For instance,

Hetherington said, "As obviously destructive as conflict is to all involved in this dilemma, it was surprising to discover that six years after divorce, 20 to 25 percent of our couples were engaged in just such conflictual behavior; former spouses would make nasty comments about each other, seek to undermine each other's relationship with the child, and fight openly in front of the child. Aside from being damaging, constant put-downs of the other parent may backfire, producing resentment and a spirited defense of the criticized parent by the child. . . . Conflictual co-parenting distresses children and undermines their well-being, and it makes parents unhappy, too. They feel guilty about fighting in front of the children, but their preoccupation with their anger and lingering resentment makes it difficult for them to begin focusing on a new, more fulfilling life and on the pain they are causing their children" (Hetherington and Kelly, 2002, page 138).

Elissa P. Benedek, M.D., and Diane H. Schetky, M.D.

Although Elissa Benedek and Diane Schetky did not conduct systematic research regarding parental alienation, they described the phenomenon in a 1985 article, "Custody and Visitation: Problems and Perspectives." They explained how some divorcing parents encourage their children to get caught up in the conflicts between the parents. For example, "[The overly anxious parent] mistrusts the former spouse and may transmit this anxiety to the child, causing the child to feel that he or she will not be safe while visiting the other parent." Also, "[The hostile, vindictive parent] may pressure the child to take sides, causing him to feel guilty about visiting the other parent. In the extreme, this may lead to brainwashing. . . . Very young children . . . may be particularly susceptible to brainwashing and come to believe that the horrible things one parent says about the other are true" (Benedek and Schetky, 1985b).

5. Parental alienation is a valid concept. There has been considerable qualitative and quantitative research regarding parental alienation and PAS.

The two primary forms of research in the social sciences are qualitative research and quantitative research. In qualitative research, data are collected usually in the form of descriptions from systematic observations, from which conclusions are drawn. In the quantitative process, data are collected in the form of empirical values or numbers and analyzed statistically, from which conclusions are drawn. Both approaches are acceptable methods of conducting research, each with its advantages and disadvantages (Golafshani, 2003). Qualitative research is used to deeply explore newer subject areas that require the generation of hypotheses. After qualitative research is conducted, the hypotheses can be tested through quantitative research. Much research regarding parental alienation has been conducted using the qualitative method and is discussed in this book, primarily with regard to the validity of parental alienation as a concept. Quantitative research has also been conducted and is discussed in this book, primarily with regard to the prevalence of parental alienation and the reliability of criteria to identify PAS.

Grounded Theory Method

Glaser and Strauss (1967) introduced social researchers to a method of conducting research called the Grounded Theory Method (GTM). Strauss et al. (2007) elaborated on the concepts and techniques of GTM. Babbie (2007) explained GTM as a four-step process. First, incidents or cases are observed and notes made. The notes from these incidents or cases are compared and similarities or differences noted, through what is referred to as comparative analysis. A phenomenon may be observed and described, which later becomes a conceptual theory. In the second step of the process, relationships among concepts are noted and integrated into categories based on their properties. In the third step of the process, continuing with comparative analysis, the researcher may further clarify the concepts. Perhaps some initial relationships deemed irrelevant are discarded. Categories may be reduced, clarifying and creating a simple, well-defined theory. In the fourth and final step of the process, the researcher puts his findings into a written report.

The process by which PAS was discovered, identified, and defined is an example of the GTM of social research, which constituted very extensive qualitative research. Richard Gardner and others were in a position to systematically observe the children of divorced parents, primarily through child custody evaluations. These mental health professionals took descriptive notes on their observations during each evaluation. These notes were the basis for subsequent reports, used to assist in treatment and/or custody decisions. The notes and reports are the equivalent of descriptive observations, that is, qualitative data. Similarities among these evaluations were noted through comparative analysis, which resulted in the development of a new theory. Gardner and others observed–while conducting child custody evolutions in the context of high-conflict divorces–a pattern in which children rejected without justification a previously loved parent. Gardner and others theorized the rejection was occurring at the hands of one of the parents, whom Gardner named the "alienating parent." Gardner gave this unwarranted rejection, a theoretical concept, the name "parental alienation syndrome" and identified eight symptoms as indicators of PAS. Gardner and others then reported in writing their findings on the phenomenon of PAS, which are discussed in the next section of this book. Gardner and other practitioners and researchers of parental alienation followed the GTM method of social research. Some of these mental health professionals did not initially set out to conduct research, but that is not a reason to discount their findings and observations. History is full of discoveries by those who accidently came upon something new or unknown.

Triangulation

Social researchers validate their work through an approach called triangulation or, more specifically, methodological triangulation. Methodological triangulation involves using different types of research methods to study a particular phenomenon. Researchers may use different qualitative methods or different quantitative methods or both.

Todd D. Jick studied this topic extensively. Jick (1979) said that different methods should be used as complementary approaches rather than as rivals. He also indicated that if the different methods reach similar conclusions, it improves the validity of the research. There are several ways to achieve methodological triangulation, such as: one researcher using two or more research techniques and two or more researchers conducting research separately using the same type of research technique. Jick noted that the use of triangulation in the social sciences is traced back to the work of Campbell and Fiske (1959) who developed the idea of "multiple operationism." It was argued that more than one method should be used in the validation process. This was to ensure that the variance reflected that of the trait and not of the method. Kraemer and her colleagues presented the same argument regarding psychiatric diagnoses. They said, "Validity is difficult to establish since it requires a criterion or 'gold standard' for the presence of the disorder that is seldom available in psychiatry. Generally, the best that can be done is to challenge validity in a variety of ways using a variety of criteria. Each challenge survived gives greater assurance of validity" (Kraemer et al., 2004).

Research regarding PAS–summarized later in this book–is a good example of methodological triangulation. Numerous mental health practitioners and researchers used different qualitative and quantitative methods to study the phenomenon of parental alienation, and they agreed that parental alienation exists and is a valid concept. Specifically, the components of methodological triangulation regarding parental alienation and PAS include the following: extensive observations of one clinician, Richard Gardner; contemporaneous, independent observations by several other clinicians and research groups; the application of Gardner's definition of PAS by other researchers to a wide variety of subjects; the recognition of parental alienation and PAS in many countries; quantitative reliability studies; and quantitative prevalence studies.

6. Parental alienation is a valid concept. In the 1980s and 1990s, parental alienation was described independently by at least six researchers or groups of researchers in the U.S.

A concept is a mental representation with meaning, and a valid concept refers to one for which there is general agreement regarding the meaning or definition of the concept. For example, is the term parental alienation a valid mental representation of the condition that Gardner defined as "a disturbance in which children were preoccupied with deprecation and criticism of a parent–denigration that is unjustified and/or exaggerated" (Gardner, 1992a, page 59)? One way to answer this question is to see whether various professional observers independently collected similar data and arrived at the same conclusions.

In the case of parental alienation, divorce researchers have consistently identified a portion of children of divorce who become alienated from one parent for no apparent reason, that is, the alienation was not due to abuse or neglect by the rejected parent. At least six individuals or research groups working independently during the 1980s and 1990s identified children of separated or divorced parents who were severely alienated from one parent without apparent justification.

Judith Wallerstein, Ph.D., and Colleagues

In 1976, Judith Wallerstein and Joan B. Kelly, Ph.D., both psychologists, identified a clinical phenomenon they called "pathological alignment," which sometimes occurred in their sample of divorcing families (Wallerstein and Kelly, 1976).

In 1980, Wallerstein and Kelly published *Surviving the Break-up: How Children and Parents Cope with Divorce.* In this important book, the authors described their landmark, long-term study of 60 community families of divorce from Northern California. Wallerstein and Kelly related that some children of divorced parents became aligned with one parent against the other. These children vehemently refused contact with one parent and appeared to be unreasonably allied with the other. The authors referred to an alliance between a narcissistically enraged parent and a particularly vulnerable older child or adolescent, who "were faithful and valuable battle allies in efforts to hurt and punish the other parent. Not infrequently, they turned on the parent they had loved and been very close to prior to the marital separation" (Wallerstein and Kelly, 1980, page 77).

In 1989, Judith Wallerstein and Sandra Blakeslee published a follow-up book, *Second Chances: Men, Women, and Children a Decade After Divorce.* The authors did not use the term "parental alienation," but they vividly related how court-ordered visitation can "be entangled with Medea-like rage." They said, "A woman betrayed by her husband is deeply opposed to the fact that her children must visit him every other weekend. . . . She cannot stop the visit, but she can plant seeds of doubt—'Do not trust your father'—in the children's minds and thus punish her ex-husband via the children. She does this consciously or unconsciously, casting the seeds of doubt by the way she acts and the questions she asks. . . . Fathers in similar circumstances make use of techniques congenial to them, often conveying to the boy or girl that the mother is depraved and dangerous" (Wallerstein and Blakeslee, 1989, page 197).

Richard Gardner, M.D.

During the 1970s and early 1980s, Richard Gardner, a child and adolescent psychiatrist, was called upon to conduct child custody evaluations, primarily in the New York City area. As a custody evaluator, Gardner was in a position to make observations, a role that was limited to those few mental health professionals who did similar types of work. As Gardner conducted custody evaluations, wrote reports, and prepared to testify in court, he made notes of his observations. In the process of collecting and organizing the descriptions of what he observed, Gardner was conducting qualitative research on the phenomenon of parental alienation.

Drawing upon these observations, Gardner introduced in 1985 the term "parental alienation syndrome" for a type of emotional child abuse almost exclusively seen in separated and divorced families engaged in custody disputes. Gardner said, "The parental alienation syndrome (PAS) is a disorder that arises primarily in the context of child custody disputes. Its primary manifestation is the child's campaign of denigration against the parent, a campaign that has no justification. The disorder results from the combination of indoctrination by the alienating parent and the child's own contributions to the vilification of the alienated parent" (Gardner, 1985).

As he continued to conduct custody evaluations and collect observational data, Gardner defined eight behaviors or symptoms as indicating the presence of PAS. These behaviors–primarily manifested by children caught between parents seeking custody during a high conflict divorce–consisted of the following: the campaign of denigration; weak, frivolous and absurd rationalizations for the deprecation; lack of ambivalence; the "independent-thinker" phenomenon; reflexive support of the preferred parent in the parental conflict; absence of guilt over cruelty to and/or exploitation of the alienated parent; presence of borrowed scenarios; and spread of animosity to the extended family of the alienated parent (Gardner, 1992a, pages 63–82).

Gardner emphasized that in PAS, the child's denigration of the alienated parent is not justified. The child's fear of the alienated parent is greatly out of proportion to anything the alienated parent did. Gardner said, "When true parental abuse and/or neglect are present, the child's animosity may be justified, and so the parental alienation syndrome explanation for the child's hostility is not applicable"

(Gardner, 1998b).

Gardner identified hundreds of children with this condition. He thought the dramatic increase in the prevalence of this condition occurred because in the late 1970s, it became much more common for fathers to seek custody of their children and for courts to order joint custodial arrangements. This created a climate in which parents would induce alienation in order to gain the upper hand in court and foil the other parent's claim for custody or visitation. Also, some jurisdictions made it easier to obtain a divorce, thus increasing the rate of divorce. Having observed the behaviors and symptoms of PAS on numerous occasions, Gardner wrote about his observations related to this topic in about 20 articles and four books (Gardner, 1987a, 1992a, 2001b; Gardner et al., 2006).

Leona Kopetski, MSSW

During the 1970s and 1980s, Leona Kopetski, a social worker, conducted child custody evaluations in Colorado. At the time, she was unaware of the work of Richard Gardner and the research of Stanley Clawar and Brynne Rivlin. In describing the phenomenon of "Parent Alienation Syndrome," Kopetski said, "Alienating parents (who should know better) and their children (who cannot be expected to know better) sometimes share a common delusion that *one* and *only one* other human being, namely the alienating parent, can provide the child with the relationship necessary for psychological survival" (Kopetski, 1998a). She also pointed out, "Parent alienation is not a gender-determined syndrome. Either the mother or father can alienate; either can be alienated" (Kopetski, 1998b). Kopetski and her team identified 84 cases of severe alienation out of 413 court-ordered evaluations conducted between 1976 and 1990 (Kopetski, 1998a, 1998b, 2006). Kopetski wrote descriptions of her observations in an effort to assist other evaluators. Kopetski's own work led her "independently to conclusions that were remarkably similar to Gardner's conclusions regarding the characteristics of the syndrome" (Kopetski, 1998a).

Stanley S. Clawar, Ph.D., C.C.S., and Brynne V. Rivlin, M.S.S.

In 1991, Stanley Clawar, a sociologist, and Brynne Rivlin, a social worker, who both conducted child custody evaluations, published a study through the American Bar Association titled *Children Held Hostage*. An increase in child custody fights passing through the family court system created a concern for how to better manage the conflict. In their research, Clawar and Rivlin followed 700 counseling cases over a 12-year period (apparently from the mid 1970s to the late 1980s), primarily in Pennsylvania. Clawar and Rivlin documented their observations over the course of their study, from which they made conclusions. They found that in about 80 percent of the cases, there was some element of parental programming in an effort to implant false and negative ideas about the other parent with the intention of turning the child against that other parent. Their work focused on emotional issues, persistent programming, and brainwashing, which sometimes resulted in severe parental alienation (Clawar and Rivlin, 1991).

Janet R. Johnston, Ph.D., and Colleagues

In 1985, Janet R. Johnston, a sociologist, Linda E. G. Campbell, Ph.D., and Sharon S. Mayes, Ph.D., reported the "distress and symptomatic behavior of 44 children, aged 6–12 years, . . . who were the subject of post-separation and divorce disputes over their custody and care." The authors described six primary responses of these children to their parents: "strong alliance," "alignment," "loyalty conflict," "shifting allegiances," "acceptance of both" with "avoidance of preferences," and "rejection of both." The authors' definition of "strong alliance" was "a strong, consistent, overt (publicly stated) verbal and behavioral preference for one parent together with rejection and denigration of the other. It is accompanied by affect that is clearly hostile, negative and unambivalent." Of the 44 children studied, 7 (16%) manifested this response (Johnston et al., 1985). It is notable that Gardner described "parental alienation syndrome" and Johnston and her colleagues described children with a "strong alliance" in the same year. They apparently were talking about the same phenomenon in different groups of subjects.

In 1993, Janet Johnston reported on two studies "of divorcing families who represent the more ongoing and entrenched disputes over custody and visitation." Together, the two studies involved 140 divorcing parents disputing the custody and visitation of 175 children. These families were referred from family courts in the San Francisco Bay

Area for counseling and mediation between 1982 and 1990. Some of these children demonstrated "strong alignment" with one parent, which meant: "The child consistently denigrated and rejected the other parent. Often, this was accompanied by an adamant refusal to visit, communicate, or have anything to do with the rejected parent." Although Johnston's research was undertaken independently of Gardner, she observed, "Strong alignments are probably most closely related to the behavioral phenomenon Gardner referred to as parental alienation syndrome. . ." (Johnston, 1993).

In 1997, Janet Johnston and Vivienne Roseby published *In the Name of the Child,* which addressed the assessment and treatment of high-conflict divorcing families. In the chapter on "Parental Alignments and Alienation among Children of High-Conflict Divorce," they say, "Most children and adolescents of divorce are eager to have an ongoing relationship with both of their parents, and most are pained by loyalty conflicts and the fear that they might have to choose one parent and lose the other. A minority of children, however, will become enmeshed in the parental conflict to such a degree that they are said to be aligned with one parent and alienated from the other" (Johnston and Roseby, 1997, page 193). A second edition of this book was recently published (Johnston et al., 2009).

In 1998, Vivienne Roseby and Janet Johnston explained rather eloquently how parental alienation comes about. In a book chapter with a dramatic title, "Children of Armageddon," they said, "A central problem in high-conflict divorce and protracted custody disputes involves the narcissistic vulnerability of the divorcing parties. . . . The other parent is seen as irrelevant, irresponsible or even dangerous, whereas the self is seen as the essential, responsible, and safe caretaker. These parents tend to selectively perceive and distort the child's concerns regarding the other parent. For example, if a vulnerable woman has experienced her ex-spouse as emotionally neglectful, she expects him to be neglectful with her child; if the child comes back upset or depressed after spending time with the father, the mother attributes the difficulty solely to the father's lack of care. . . . In this way, vulnerable parents overidentify with elements of the child's emotional response that remind them of their own experience with the ex-spouse and confirm the other parent's 'badness.' Thus, such a mother will amplify and distort her perception of the child's sadness and anxiety, and run the risk of distorting the child's reality testing about his or her own feelings and ideas" (Roseby and Johnston, 1998).

In 2001, Joan Kelly and Janet Johnston critiqued Gardner's definition of PAS and proposed an alternative framework for classifying
alienated children. Although Janet Johnston and Joan Kelly agree that
parental alienation is a real phenomenon, they do not agree with the
concept of parental alienation *syndrome.* Their work is sometimes
referred to as the "reformulation" of PAS, which meant that the focus
of the assessment should be on the child, not on the parent as embod-
ied in the concept of PAS. Kelly and Johnston believe that parental
alienation is not necessarily caused primarily by an alienating parent.
Rather, they discussed alienation as a result of interrelated systemic
processes with contributing factors within the environment, within
each parent, and in the child to "create and/or consolidate alienation"
of a child from a once-loved parent (Kelly and Johnston, 2001).

Although they started with somewhat different assumptions about
etiology, both Gardner and Kelly and Johnston apparently identified
the same group of children. For example, Gardner thought that PAS
consisted of eight specific symptoms. In their alternative framework,
Kelly and Johnston listed almost the identical symptoms as features of
what they called the "alienated child." For instance, Gardner's list
included "weak, absurd, or frivolous rationalizations for the deprecation" of a parent; Kelly and Johnston's list included "trivial or false reasons used to justify hatred" (Kelly and Johnston, 2001). Also, Kelly and
Johnston defined an alienated child as "one who expresses freely and
persistently unreasonable negative feelings and beliefs (such as anger,
hatred, rejection and/or fear) toward a parent that are significantly dis-
proportionate to the child's actual experience with that parent."
Although these authors do not agree with the concept of parental
alienation *syndrome,* they endorse the basic premise of parental alienation, that some children ally with one parent against the other parent
in the absence of abuse or neglect.

Johnston's definition of an "alienated child" is almost exactly the
same as our concept of "parental alienation." We also agree with
Johnston's statement that "it is important to differentiate *alienated* children (who persistently refuse visitation and stridently express unrealistic negative views and feelings) from other children who also resist
contact with a parent after separation but for a variety of expectable
reasons, including *normal developmental preferences* for one parent, *alignments* that are reactions to the specific circumstances of the divorce,

and *estrangement* from a parent who has been neglectful or abusive" (Johnston, 2005, emphasis in original text). Furthermore, we agree that there are various routes to becoming an alienated child, as there are various causes of parental alienation. Since our definitions and opinions seemed highly congruent, we have encouraged Janet Johnston since October 2008 to participate with us in developing this proposal for DSM-5 and ICD-11; she has declined our invitations.

One of Johnston's reasons for not supporting either "the alienated child" or "parental alienation" as a diagnostic entity is that sometimes it is hard to tell the difference between alienation (which is unjustified) and estrangement (which is justified because of the rejected parent's neglectful or abusive behaviors). However, in their own research, Johnston and her colleagues studied the records of separating and divorced families and were able to tell the difference between cases in which allegations of abuse were substantiated and those in which allegations of abuse were not substantiated. They based their determinations on the type of information and documents that are commonly collected in both clinical and forensic evaluations–such as interviews of family members, observations of the interactions between parents and children, information from collateral professionals and other individuals, and written documentation provided by attorneys and parents (Johnston, Lee, Olesen, and Walters, 2005).

Barry Bricklin, Ph.D.

From the mid 1960s to the present, Barry Bricklin, a psychologist, has conducted child custody research, which was published in book chapters and books (for example, Bricklin, 1995), as well as in peer-reviewed journals and law reviews. Thousands of children and their parents were evaluated and in some cases there have been seven years of follow-up data. Bricklin studied children who voiced strongly-worded verbal opinions about parents that were inconsistent with other information. In his research, Bricklin called this phenomenon Not-Based-On-Actual-Interactions (NBOAI). That is, a child made verbal statements that were likely not based on his or her actual interactions with the person being spoken about, but rather on what the child had been manipulated, bribed, or coerced into saying and possibly believing. Children were most susceptible to these manipulations when they viewed the parent doing the manipulating as needing help to survive psychologically or needing retribution for some, usually imagined, wrong.

Bricklin identified four categories of NBOAI, one of which strongly resembled the parental alienation syndrome as that entity was being discussed in the prevailing psychological literature. The signs for this category of NBOAI were described as follows:

1. The child expressed a strong favorable verbal opinion of the parent he or she wished to live with, and a strong negative verbal opinion of the parent he or she "never wanted to see again."
2. On a test in which it was consciously obvious to the child whom he or she would be endorsing on each test item, all or almost all of the endorsements were for the favored parent by huge and statistically rare margins.
3. On a nonverbal test where it was not consciously obvious what the statistically-based responses meant, there were several endorsements for the nonfavored parent.
4. When the child was asked to give sense-based real-life examples of negative endorsements, these examples were mostly trivial or downright irrelevant to the issues supposedly involved.

It is important to note that these six groups of clinicians and researchers—working during the same period of time—independently identified the same phenomenon. This is very strong evidence that the consistent pattern of behaviors, which we are calling parental alienation, really exists as a distinct clinical entity.

7. Parental alienation is a valid concept. After PAS was formally defined by Richard Gardner, many mental health researchers applied that definition to study children of high-conflict divorces. These researchers verified that Gardner's definition could be used to identify groups of children who fulfilled the diagnostic criteria of PAS.

One way to establish the external validity and ecological validity of a concept is to apply the criteria for the concept to other samples to see if similar individuals are identified. Converging results from multiple samples allows for more generalization and strengthens both external and ecological validity. After the criteria for PAS were widely published and understood—for example, through *The Parental Alienation Syndrome: A Guide for Mental Health and Legal Professionals* (Gardner, 1992a)—researchers applied these criteria to totally separate samples of children of divorced parents. They found that Gardner's criteria allowed them to identify parents and children with a particular cluster of symptoms, which we call parental alienation.

Most of the research discussed in this section of the book was conducted in the U.S. and published in English. See Section 9 for a discussion of many research studies that were conducted and published in other countries. The research cited in this section was either published in a peer-reviewed journal or was a dissertation written for a graduate degree in psychology or a related field. Dissertation research is guided by committees composed of experts at the doctoral level, which is analogous to peer review. The following research studies are in chronological order.

John Dunne, M.D., and Marsha Hedrick, Ph.D.

In 1994, John Dunne and Marsha Hedrick, who worked in Seattle, published a study involving 16 cases of severe parental alienation which were very resistant to clinical intervention. Using Gardner's criteria for PAS, these authors found that the syndrome can occur without reference to the length of the relationship prior to the separation and can occur immediately following separation or not until many years after the divorce. They also found that it can occur throughout the age range, from very young children to teenagers who had previously enjoyed a lengthy positive post-divorce relationship with the alienated parent. In their study, PAS could involve all the children in a family or only one. Although the alienating parent was most often the custodial mother, alienation by non-custodial parents, usually fathers, also occurred. Dunne and Hedrick thought that the motivations of the alienating parents were often out of their consciousness or colored in socially acceptable ways (Dunne and Hedrick, 1994).

Larry Nicholas, Ph.D.

In 1997, Larry Nicholas, a forensic psychologist practicing in California, reported on a survey of 21 custody evaluators. Nicholas

Severe Parental Alienation Resolves—After Parents Remarry
John Dunne, M.D., Seattle, Washington

This was a very unusual case of parental alienation, in which the child eventually enjoyed a good relationship with both parents. Dr. Dunne said he treated a little boy, Matthew, whose parents divorced when he was 3 years old. After the divorce, Matthew and his mother moved to the Seattle area to be closer to the mother's extended family. Matthew's mother said she wanted to get away from "the father's anger."

When Matthew was 6 years old, Dr. Dunne treated him for about one year because Matthew was very resistant to visiting his father, who lived in another state. Matthew refused to see his father even if the visitation were to occur in Seattle. The mother nominally supported Matthew's visitation with his father, but she did not want to "pressure" or "distress" the child. During the entire year of treatment, no contact ever occurred between Matthew and his father.

Many years later, a young man came to Dr. Dunne's office, introduced himself, and said that he had been a patient when he was a little boy. Matthew told Dr. Dunne that when he was 12 years old, his parents started corresponding. When he was 15, over his strenuous objections, he and his mother moved to his father's city and his parents soon remarried. At the time of the remarriage, Matthew said he still disliked his father and avoided him. However, by the time he was 16, Matthew reported that he had a very good relationship with his father as well as with his mother. None of this occurred with any professional intervention.

Dr. Dunne said, "The point of the case is that the alienation resolved only after the parents reconciled, and even then with some delay."

---

sought to determine whether there was a cluster of identifiable attitudes and behaviors in the alienating parent, the target parent, and the child, which could be said to constitute a syndrome as Gardner suggested. Parent alienating behaviors were found to be highly correlated with children's alienation symptoms and vice versa. There were no significant correlations between the child's alienation symptoms and eight of ten target parent characteristics. Significant correlations were found, however, between child alienation symptoms and two target parent items: temporarily giving up on the child and becoming irritated and angry with the child for exhibiting the alienating behaviors. The findings of Nicholas' survey support Gardner's contention that the core dynamic in PAS is between the alienating parent and child, and that the target parent's behavior is much less likely to be a major contributing factor (Nicholas, 1997).

Deirdre Conway Rand, Ph.D., and Colleagues

Between 1997 and 2005, Deirdre Rand, a forensic psychologist practicing in California, published "The Spectrum of Parental Alienation Syndrome" in three parts. Part I discussed social changes, the etiology of PAS, and the behaviors of parents who induce PAS (Rand, 1997a). Rand reviewed the descriptions of parental alienation and PAS by Gardner (1987a, 1989a, 1992a), Clawar and Rivlin (1991), Turkat (1994, 1995), and several other authors. Part II described the behaviors of children after PAS had been introduced (Rand, 1997b). She also discussed other aspects of PAS, such as the contribution of the targeted parent, the involvement of third parties, and the response of the legal system to PAS. In Part III, Deirdre Rand and Randy Rand, Ed.D., joined Leona Kopetski, MSSW (Rand et al., 2005). They sought to evaluate methods to therapeutically interrupt PAS in 45 custody evaluations and present the results of their research. Deirdre Rand has written another article (Rand, in press) which discusses "critics of parental alienation syndrome and the politics of science."

Jeffrey C. Siegel, Ph.D., and Joseph S. Langford, Ph.D.

In 1998, Jeffrey Siegel and Joseph Langford published an important paper, "MMPI-2 Validity Scales and Suspected Parental Alienation Syndrome." The authors said, "The present study is an attempt to gain understanding of parents who engage in alienating tactics through a statistical examination of their MMPI-2 validity scales." The study involved 34 female subjects who completed the MMPI-2 in the course of child custody evaluations. Of the total, 16 subjects met the criteria for classification as PAS parents; 18 were considered non-PAS parents. Siegel and Langford concluded, "The hypothesis was confirmed for K and F scales, indicating that PAS parents are more likely to complete MMPI-2 questions in a defensive manner, striving to appear as flawless as possible. It was concluded that parents who engage in alienating behaviors are more likely than other parents to use the psychological defenses of denial and projection, which are associated with this validity scale pattern" (Siegel and Langford, 1998).

Jodi Stoner-Moskowitz, Psy.D.

In 1998, Jodi Stoner-Moskowitz completed a dissertation that examined the relationship of children's self-concept to four types of family structure, Intact, Divorced, High Conflict, and Alienated families. Stoner-Moskowitz, using Gardner's definition of PAS to define the Alienated families, examined 141 children of divorced parents. Stoner-Moskowitz found that children in all four groups had diminished self-concept; divorce conflict was inversely correlated with self-concept (Stoner-Moskowitz, 1998).

Despina Vassiliou, Psy.D.

In 2001, Despina Vassiliou and Glenn Cartwright published a small, qualitative study involving five fathers and one mother who had experienced PAS. The data were collected via semistructured, open-ended interviews to determine if there were shared characteristics among alienated families, common issues in the marital conflicts that contributed to the marriage dissolution, the nature of the participants' reports of alienation, similarities in the experience of alienation, and what things a lost parent might do differently. Vassiliou observed that a tactic used by the alienating parent is that of denigration aimed at the targeted parent and that children aligned with the alienating parent will join in the process. Overall, Vassiliou found that there are several possible attributes that may be precursors or indicators of PAS (Vassiliou and Cartwright, 2001).

In 2005, Vassiliou completed a dissertation for graduate school. The purpose of this research was to find identifiable characteristic of PAS. Vassiliou examined targeted parents' experiences with the legal system as their cases passed through the family court. Vassiliou also compared PAS and false allegations of abuse, and she sought to identify similarities and differences and examine possible relationships between the two. Vassiliou found that interference in visitation was a common tactic used for those inflicting PAS. Also, she found that all participants left with negative perceptions of lawyers, judges, and the family court system (Vassiliou, 2005).

Janelle Burrill, Ph.D.

In 2001, Janelle Burrill published significant research regarding PAS. Burrill examined 30 families with 59 children, who were referred to her for evaluation, therapy, or mediation. The selection criteria for her study were intractable parental conflict and custody disputes, manifested by at least two court appearances during a 24-month period commencing January 1998. Using the Gardner criteria for identifying and categorizing PAS, Burrill was able to sort the parents–based on their PAS symptoms–into the mild, moderate, and severe categories. She was able to sort the children–based on their PAS symptoms–into the mild, moderate, and severe categories. Burrill compared the number of symptoms manifested by the parents and the children in these various groups. She found a correlation between the parents' symptoms and the children's symptoms. She found a correlation between the alienating parents' behaviors and the child's negative behaviors toward the alienated parent. Burrill concluded, "The data from this study appear to support Dr. Gardner's observations of PAS published in 1985. . . . In its severe form, PAS is more distinctive than the mild form. PAS is destructive to a child's relationship with the alienated parent. Severe PAS can be irreversible in its effects. Severe PAS is destructive irrespective of the gender of the alienating parent. Children's negative behaviors towards the alienating parent increase in severity as the negative behaviors and hostility of the alienating parent increases. The results of this data are significant" (Burrill, 2001, page 78).

Kristen Marie Carey, Psy.D.

In 2003, Kristen Marie Carey completed a dissertation for graduate school. She identified subjects in the San Francisco Bay area who had some degree of parental alienation. Of the ten subjects, eight were found to have been affected by PAS upon the divorce of their parents, and Carey was able to categorize them as mild, moderate, or severe based on Gardner's criteria. The two remaining subjects manifested some degree of parental alienation, but not PAS. It is notable that only six of the ten subjects had recovered their relationship with the alienated parent. Although her sample size was small, Carey confirmed the existence of the phenomenon of PAS (Carey, 2003).

Jean Andrew Deters, Psy.D.

In 2003, Jean Andrew Deters completed a dissertation for graduate school. Deters' research was based on the assumption that the phenomenon of PAS existed. He sought to find methods for courts to deal with high-conflict divorce and ongoing parental alienation. He described how models based on "parent coordinating" would help courts deal with these issues (Deters, 2003). Since Deters conducted the research for his dissertation, many states have adopted the role of "parenting coordinator" to help parents communicate in a constructive manner, reduce the conflict, and follow the court-ordered parenting plan.

Cynthia Raso, M.A.

In 2004, Cynthia Raso completed a dissertation for graduate school, a qualitative study regarding the long-term effects of PAS. Raso examined eleven subjects who were self-identified as victims of PAS. After conducting detailed interviews, Raso found, "The more severe the PAS, the more likely the child will develop externalizing problems (drugs and alcohol, early sexual and promiscuous sexual activity and disciplinary problems at school). . . . The more severe the PAS, the more likely the child will develop internalizing problems (issues with trust, intimacy, and commitment). . . . The more severe the PAS, the more likely the child, if she/he becomes a parent and goes through a divorce, will handle his/her divorce differently from the way his/her parents did. . . . The more severe the PAS, the more likely the non-custodial parent-child relationship will be damaged for life." Raso concluded that PAS has detrimental effects for the alienated child and that the effects continue into adulthood (Raso, 2004).

Luisa Pederson Machuca, M.S.

In 2005, Luisa Pederson Machuca completed a dissertation for graduate school. Machuca used Gardner's definition and eight symptoms of PAS. In this research, Machuca evaluated a test instrument for determining presence of PAS. She examined 329 students from Anchorage, Alaska, who were divided into two groups, parents divorced and parents non-divorced. Machuca assessed which of the eight symptoms of PAS contributed to the occurrence of PAS; four were identified for mothers and three for fathers. Machuca concluded her test instrument was valid to measure the presence of PAS (Machuca, 2005). It is notable that Machuca identified some subjects as having PAS, so her research confirmed the existence of the concept of PAS.

Amy J. L. Baker, Ph.D., and Colleagues

In 2006, Amy J. L. Baker, Ph.D., and Douglas Darnall, Ph.D., completed a study of targeted parents who were asked to describe in detail the behaviors exhibited by the alienating parents. Independent coding that achieved inter-rater reliability identified the most common strategies. These strategies were consistent with those identified by adults who as children were turned against one parent by the other (Baker and Darnall, 2006).

In 2007, Baker and Darnall published a survey in which 97 targeted parents were asked to rate the severity of the alienating parent's alienation strategies (naïve, active, obsessed) as well as the degree of the child's alienation (mild, moderate, severe). Although 90 percent of the parents were rated as obsessed (defined as, "S/he has a mission to destroy the relationship between the targeted parent and the child."), only 44 percent of the children were rated as severely alienated (defined as, "Your child professes to want nothing to do with you. Visitation is minimal if at all."). In other words, not all children exposed to alienating behavior succumb to the pressure to choose sides. The primary purpose of this study was to determine the extent to which targeted parents describe their alienated children's behavior as being consistent with the eight behavioral manifestations of PAS as identified by Richard Gardner. Although this was borne out in general, it was also discovered that even the most alienated child will present some "crack in the armor" which can be used as a window of opportunity by targeted parents for countering the alienation (Baker and Darnall, 2007).

In 2007, Baker published the results of an empirical investigation into the beliefs and practices of custody evaluators. Baker found that over 70 percent of survey respondents reported that they "very much" believed that it was possible for a parent to turn a child against the other parent in the absence of abuse, neglect, or abandonment (essentially a restatement of the core idea of PAS), and 75 percent said that they "very much" thought it was important to assess the presence of parental alienation in custody evaluations (Baker, 2007a).

Also in 2007, Baker published a book describing the results of in-depth interviews with adults who believed that when they were children they had been turned against one parent by the other. These data presented the first look at the phenomenon of parental alienation from the perspective of the children who lived through it and provided compelling validation that parents are able to emotionally manipulate children to reject a parent that they would otherwise have no reason or desire to reject. The study also provided harrowing accounts of the negative lifelong impact of this experience for the child victims (Baker, 2007b).

A very recent collaborative study between the Vincent J. Fontana Center for Child Protection and New York University revealed that about 28 percent of adults in a community sample (i.e., not selected because of a precondition related to divorce or custody) reported that when they were children one parent tried to turn them against the other. These data are striking in that a significant portion of the sample was probably raised in an intact family. Not surprisingly, the proportion who reported that they had been exposed to parental alienation (defined in the study as one parent trying to turn the child against the other parent) was higher in the subsample of individuals who had been raised by a stepparent, at 44 percent. Thus, it would fair to estimate that in 40 percent to 80 percent of all divorcing families, one parent exhibits parental alienation tactics, at least periodically (Baker, 2010).

Kathleen M. Reay, Ph.D.

In 2007, Kathleen M. Reay completed a dissertation for graduate school. Reay conducted a quantitative study designed to answer the following question: "Do adult children of divorce with different levels of PAS show corresponding levels of psychological distress." Reay used Gardner's concept of PAS and the symptoms of PAS to conduct her study. She collected data from 150 adults from a Canadian community, who had been selected based on specified criteria. Based on responses to questionnaires, Reay determined the level of PAS for each subject as mild, moderate, or severe. Next, Reay used a separate questionnaire to determine each respondent's present psychological distress. Upon analyzing the data for correlations, Reay found, "As the level of PAS increased, so did the measurable level of psychological distress." Reay concluded that her research lends support to Richard Gardner's theory of PAS, with a lifetime of mental health issues observed to occur for those victimized by PAS. Reay thought her data analysis supported the scientific validity of PAS (Reay, 2007).

Melissa Colarossi, M.A.

In 2007, Melissa Colarossi completed a dissertation for graduate school. She conducted a small qualitative study regarding the impact of marital separation and divorce on individuals. Colarossi examined twelve subjects and found two cases of PAS. She found that the two individuals who had experienced PAS manifested sadness because their ex-wives were making sure they would not be able to spend time with their children. Colarossi noted that alienating parents strive to cut off contact between the targeted parent and the children (Colarossi, 2007).

Robert Gordon, Ph.D., and Colleagues

In 2008, Robert Gordon, Ronald Stoffey, and Jennifer Bottinelli published important research regarding the use of objective psychological testing–the Minnesota Multiphasic Personality Inventory–2 (MMPI-2)–with families involved in custody disputes. The authors collected the MMPI-2 results from the parents who had been seen in 158 court-ordered custody evaluations. Of these cases, 76 were PAS cases and 82 were custody cases without PAS (controls). The subjects were identified as alienating parent, target parent and control parent. Two different MMPI-2 indexes were used to measure primitive defenses: $L + K - F$ and $(L + Pa + Sc) - (Hy + Pt)$. The authors found that mothers and fathers who were alienators had higher scores (in the clinical range), indicating primitive defenses such as splitting and projective identification, than control mothers and fathers (scores in the normal range). The scores of target parents were mostly similar to the scores of control parents. Overall, this study strongly supported Gardner's definition of PAS (Gordon et al., 2008).

James N. Bow, Ph.D., and Colleagues

In 2009, James N. Bow, Jonathan W. Gould, and James R. Flens published their research in which they surveyed 448 mental health and legal professionals about their knowledge of parental alienation and PAS. They found their subjects, as a group, to be knowledgeable about parental alienation and aware of the controversies regarding this topic. The authors found that on the average, their respondents had attended five conferences and read ten books or articles that addressed parental alienation (Bow et al., 2009).

8. Parental alienation is a valid concept. Despite controversies regarding terminology and etiology, the phenomenon of parental alienation is almost universally accepted by psychiatrists, psychologists, social workers, and family counselors who evaluate and treat children of high-conflict divorces.

During the 1990s and into the 2000s—after Gardner and other authors described the features of parental alienation—hundreds and perhaps thousands of mental health professionals in North America, South America, Europe, Africa, Australia, and Asia identified the same constellation of symptoms in children of parents who were embroiled in high-conflict divorces. Psychologists, psychiatrists, family counselors, and other mental health professionals have described individual cases and small groups of divorcing families that manifested the same pattern of parental alienation. This extensive literature has provided a wealth of observations regarding this phenomenon. The following citations do not constitute systematic research, but they reflect the widespread acceptance of the concept of parental alienation among mental health professionals. These articles and chapters are discussed in chronological order.

Frank S. Williams, M.D.

In 1990, Frank S. Williams, a child and adolescent psychiatrist and family therapist who practiced in Los Angeles, give the keynote address at the annual meeting of the National Council for Children's Rights in Washington, D.C. Williams' address was titled "Preventing Parentectomy Following Divorce." He said, "Parentectomy is the removal, erasure, or severe diminution of a caring parent in a child's life, following separation or divorce. Parentectomy covers a large range of parent removal from partial parentectomy, 'You may visit your Daddy or Mommy every other Sunday'; to total parentectomy, as in Parental Alienation Syndrome, described by Gardner; or complete parent absence or removal. The victims of parentectomy are the children and the parents so severed from each other's lives. A parentectomy is the most cruel infringement upon children's rights to be carried out against human children by human adults. Parentectomies are psychologically lethal to children and parents" (Williams, 1990).

Glenn F. Cartwright, Ph.D.

In 1993, Glenn F. Cartwright, a psychologist, published "Expanding the Parameters of Parental Alienation Syndrome" (Cartwright, 1993). Cartwright is a professor in the Department of Educational and Counseling Psychology at McGill University in Canada. He frequently lectures on PAS and maintains an Internet web site that provides information regarding PAS to the public. Also, Cartwright (2006) described the process by which an alienated child sometimes reconciles with a lost parent.

Ira Daniel Turkat, Ph.D.

Since 1994, Ira Daniel Turkat, a clinical psychologist practicing in Florida, has written about PAS (Turkat, 1995, 1997, 2000, 2005). He conceptualized PAS as being a feature or a condition of one of the parents, not the child. For instance, Turkat said, "In certain cases, child visitation interference is a direct result of a custodial parent suffering from a Parental Alienation Syndrome. Here, the custodial parent engages in a variety of direct and indirect methods designed to alienate the child from his or her nonresidential parent. The result is that the child becomes preoccupied with unjustified criticism and hatred of the nonresidential parent" (Turkat, 1994). Most writers have conceptualized PAS as being a feature or a condition of the child, not of the parent. Subsequently, in "Parental alienation syndrome: A review of critical issues," Turkat discussed the spectrum of PAS and the problems and difficulties faced by social researchers studying this topic (Turkat, 2002).

Carla B. Garrity, Ph.D., and Mitchell A. Baris, Ph.D.

In 1994, Carla Garrity and Mitchell Baris published *Caught in the Middle: Protecting the Children of High-Conflict Divorce*. Although not exclusively about PAS, the authors discussed that topic. They said, "Parental alienation is very real. It occurs when one parent convinces the children that the other parent is not trustworthy, lovable, or caring—in short, not a good parent. This persuasion may be consciously malicious and intended to destroy the children's relationship with the other parent. Or it may take a more insidious, even unconscious form arising from the personality issues as yet unresolved in the childhood of one parent" (Garrity and Baris, 1994, page 66). These authors introduced the concept of the parenting coordinator, who had two tasks: "(1) translating the visitation plan into a conflict-reduction plan tailored specifically to the dynamics of the divorce impasse, and (2) assisting parents to implement it on an ongoing basis" (Garrity and Baris, 1994, page 120). Parenting coordination has become an important intervention for children who manifest mild and moderate degrees of parental alienation.

William Bernet, M.D.

In 1995, William Bernet published the first edition of *Children of Divorce: A Practical Guide for Parents, Attorneys, and Therapists* (Bernet, 1995). Bernet described "parental alienation through indoctrination" (consistent with the Gardner definition of PAS) and "parental alienation without indoctrination" (when the child gravitates to one parent or the other simply to get out of the war zone of parental battles). Bernet, a child and adolescent psychiatrist, also described the phenomenon of parental alienation in an article, "Child Custody Evaluations" (Bernet, 2002) and a major reference, the *Handbook of Child and Adolescent Psychiatry* (Bernet, 1998).

Kenneth H. Waldron, Ph.D., and David E. Joanis, J.D.

In 1996, Kenneth Waldron and David Joanis described parental alienation syndrome as a family dynamic that can have long-term deleterious effects on the child because the child learns that "hostile, obnoxious behavior is acceptable in relationships and that deceit and manipulation are a normal part of relationships" (Waldron and Joanis, 1996).

Mother Says Child Fears Father, Child Disagrees
William Bernet, M.D., Nashville, Tennessee

In custody and visitation disputes, it is common for one parent to characterize the child as having extremely negative feelings toward the other parent. That happened in the case of Charles, age 6, whose parents had divorced two years previously. There were continual disagreements regarding the father's visitation schedule, and the judge ordered that Dr. Bernet conduct a forensic evaluation and make recommendations.

Charles' mother was an anxious woman who was overprotective and interpreted benign information in the most negative light. For example, when Charles displayed advanced knowledge regarding sexual activity, his mother assumed he had been sexually abused. Actually, Charles and his mother lived in a rural community where cattle and horses were bred, so he knew a lot about reproduction. Charles' mother said the boy had nightmares about his father. She said he kept a toy rubber hatchet under his pillow in case his father were to come unexpectedly into his bedroom at night. Charles' therapist agreed that the boy feared his father and should not be forced to see him. Because of the mother's and therapist's concerns, Charles had not seen his father for several months.

As part of the custody and visitation evaluation, Dr. Bernet proposed to have one meeting with Charles and his mother together and another meeting with Charles and his father together. Charles' mother opposed that plan because she thought her son would be terrified. Charles himself, however, seemed comfortable with the proposal, so Dr. Bernet arranged to see Charles and his father together. When the father entered the meeting room, the first thing Charles said was, "Daddy, where have you been? Why haven't you called me?" Then, Charles sat on his father's lap and they drew pictures together.

Charles had a mild degree of parental alienation. When he talked to his mother and his therapist, he expressed fear of his father and reluctance to have contact with his father. However, when allowed to spend time together, Charles was perfectly comfortable and enjoyed a healthy relationship with his father. This case illustrates how an anxious parent can project his or her own fears onto the child, when the child is not actually afraid of the targeted parent. It is important—when conducting an evaluation—to collect information from all involved family members, not just one side of the dispute.

J. Michael Bone, Ph.D., and Michael R. Walsh

In 1997 and 1999, J. Michael Bone (a psychotherapist and family law mediator) and Michael R. Walsh (a marital and family law lawyer) published articles regarding PAS in a legal journal in Florida. Bone and Walsh based their writings on Gardner's definition of PAS. They said, for example, "The strategies utilized by the [alienating parent] to alienate the children and the other parent vary from the most subtle to the most obvious. They all, however, have a consistent theme: any opportunity for the [alienating parent] to control access and contact or the sharing of major decisions with reference to the child is apt to be exploited" (Walsh and Bone, 1997). Bone and Walsh also identified "four very specific criteria that can be used to identify potential PAS": one parent actively blocks access or contact between the child and the absent parent; false or unfounded accusations of abuse against the absent parent; a deterioration in the relationship between the children and the absent parent following the parents' separation; the children's fear in displeasing or disagreeing with the potentially alienating parent (Bone and Walsh, 1999).

Douglas Darnall, Ph.D.

In 1998, Douglas Darnall, a clinical psychologist with over 25 years of experience, published *Divorce Casualties: Protecting Your Children from Parental Alienation,* which discussed the spectrum of parental alienation. Darnall used the term "parental alienation" for the adult behaviors and processes that cause PAS. He proposed a three-tier classification system, now in common use, that distinguishes between naïve, active and obsessed alienators. Naïve alienators make negative comments about the other parent but without serious intent to undermine the child's relationship with that parent. Their negative comments tend to be careless remarks, and, in general, naïve alienators support the child's relationship with the other parent. Active alienators are more consistent and determined in their alienating behaviors. There is an intentional desire to criticize and undermine the targeted parent. Deep down, however, active alienators realize that what they are doing is wrong and potentially harmful to the child. By contrast, obsessed alienators are determined to destroy the child's relationship with the targeted parent. Obsessed alienators are extremists. They pressure the child to adopt their own negative view of the targeted parent, put much pressure on the child to emphatically reject the targeted parent, and cannot tolerate a good relationship between the child and the targeted parent. Also, Darnall created a 49-item questionnaire to help determine the presence of behaviors that induce PAS (Darnall, 1998, pages 18–22).

The second editon of Darnall's book was called *Divorce Casualties: Understanding Parental Alienation* (Darnall, 2008). Also, Darnall and Barbara F. Steinberg, Ph.D. (2008a, 2008b), published an interesting two-part article regarding spontaneous reunification between an estranged or aliented child and a rejected parent. They reviewed 27 cases of spontaneous reunification and noted that a psychosocial crisis was frequently the motivating event that set reunification in motion. Finally, Darnall (2010) has recently published a book on the treatment of parental alienation, *Beyond Divorce Casualties: Reunifying the Alienated Family.*

Elizabeth M. Ellis, Ph.D.

In 2000, Elizabeth Ellis published *Divorce Wars: Interventions with Families in Conflict.* Ellis discussed parental alienation extensively in this book and said, "Although the term [PAS] has not gained formal acceptance by the American Psychiatric Association, it has come to be accepted by clinicians working with families involved in postdivorce conflict. Definitions for PAS have been unclear, because clinicians still confuse the child's symptoms with the parent's behavior and the qualities of the relationship between the child and the alienating parent" (Ellis, 2000, page 227). Ellis conceptualized PAS as a mild form of *folie à deux* and she proposed DSM-style criteria for its diagnosis. Ellis suggested that the diagnosis of PAS should require that the child or adolescent manifest nine of the following twelve criteria: the child maintains a delusion of being persecuted by a parent; the child uses the mechanism of splitting to reduce ambiguity; the child denies any positive feelings for the targeted parent; the attribution of negative qualities to the targeted parent may take on a quality of distortion or bizarreness; the child states "recollections" of events that occurred out of the child's presence; the child's sense of persecution by the targeted parent has the quality of a litany; the child, when faced with contact with the targeted parent, displays a reaction of extreme anxiety; the child has a dependent and enmeshed relationship with the alienating parent; the child is highly cooperative with all adults other than the targeted parent; the child views the alienating parent as a victim; the child maintains a complete lack of concern about the targeted parent; and the child's belief system is particularly rigid, fixed, and resistant to traditional methods of intervention (adapted from Ellis, 2000, pages 229–232).

Richard Warshak, Ph.D.

In 2001, Richard Warshak published *Divorce Poison,* perhaps the best known book for both professionals and the general public regarding the topic of parental alienation (Warshak, 2001a). A clinical professor at the University of Texas Southwestern Medical Center, Warshak has over 30 years of experience in evaluating and treating children, adolescents, and families. Warshak–among others–provided an explanation that we believe supports the acceptance of PAS as an official diagnosis. He said, "PAS fits a basic pattern of many psychiatric syndromes. Such syndromes denote conditions in which people who are exposed to a designated stimulus develop a certain cluster of symptoms. . . . These diagnoses carry no implication that everyone exposed to the same stimulus develops the condition, nor that similar symptoms never develop in the absence of the designated stimulus. . . . Similarly, some, but not all, children develop PAS when exposed to a parent's negative influence. Other factors, beyond the stimulus of an alienating parent, can help elucidate the etiology for any particular child" (Warshak, 2006).

Diana Mercer, J.D., and Marsha Kline Pruett, Ph.D.

In 2001, Diana Mercer and Marshal Kline Pruett published *Your Divorce Advisor: A Lawyer and a Psychologist Guide You Through the Legal and Emotional Landscape of Divorce.* Although this book is not exclusively devoted to PAS, it does address this topic. The authors said, "The field of law and psychology has created a term for when a child does not want to visit the nonresidential parent, and expresses that refusal with venom and vehemence. The child shows disregard for the parent, maybe even hatred. The term is Parental Alienation Syndrome (PAS). PAS occurs when children become allied with one parent to a degree that they refuse to have any contact with the other parent. The hatred they express often reflects the feelings of their primary parent. They become echoes of one parent's disdain for the other. This may be communicated directly to the children, until that parent cultivates negative feelings in the children that become deep-rooted and unmalleable" (Mercer and Pruett, 2001, page 256).

Philip M. Stahl, Ph.D.

In 2003, Philip M. Stahl, a psychologist who practiced in Arizona, explained that pathological alienation is caused by the attitudes and behaviors of all three parties, the aligned parent, the rejected parent, and the child. He also emphasized, "When children are caught up in the midst of this conflict and become alienated, the emotional response can be devastating to the child's development. The degree of damage to the child's psyche will vary depending on the intensity of the alienation and the age and vulnerability of the child. However, the impact is never benign because of the fact of the child's distortions and confusions" (Stahl, 2003). Stahl published extensively regarding child custody evaluations and parenting children of divorce, including three books (Stahl, 1994, 1999a, 2007).

Barbara Jo Fidler, Ph.D., and Colleagues

In 2008, Barbara Jo Fidler, Nicholas Bala, LL.M., Rachel Birnbaum, Ph.D., and Katherine Kavassalis, LL.B., published *Challenging Issues in Child Custody Assessments: A Guide for Legal and Mental Health Professionals.* Fidler and Birnbaum are mental health professionals; Bala and Kavassalis are lawyers. In the chapter titled "Understanding Child Alienation and Its Impact on Families," the authors said, "Children from separated and divorced families who vigorously resist or refuse contact with one parent frequently are referred for child custody assessments. . . . There is significant debate in the mental health and legal literature about the conceptualization and etiology of parent-child contact problems, and about the most appropriate mental health interventions and judicial remedies relating to them. Although most authors agree that the phenomenon exists, finding an appropriate name for the problem is also a subject of debate" (Fidler et al., 2008a, page 203).

Recently, Fidler and Bala (2010) published an excellent overview of the most important issues regarding parental alienation, including the differential diagnosis of contact refusal. These authors summarized the effects of alienation on children, adult children, and the rejected parent and also potential interventions and "remedies." Fidler and Bala provided a cogent list of "recommendations for practice and policy," which included the following: prevention; education and standards for professionals; early identification, screening, triage, and expedited process; detailed and unambiguous parenting plan orders; early and vigilant case management by one judge; effective enforcement of all court orders; improving professional collaboration; judicial control after a trial; further development of clinical and educational programs and interventions; better access to services; and more and better research.

Michael G. Brock, M.A., and Samuel Saks, J.D.

In 2008, Michael Brock, a forensic mental health professional in private practice, and Samuel Saks, an attorney, published *Contemporary Issues in Family Law and Mental Health*. This book was part of the American Series in Behavioral Science and Law. Although not exclusively about PAS, the authors discussed this topic. They said, "The motivation behind a pattern of alienation is not difficult to discover if one considers all the surrounding circumstances. Yet it does require mental heath professionals to undertake a thorough investigation of the situation and not merely accept the presenting parent's perspective. . . . False allegations of abuse represent the most extreme form of alienation" (Brock and Saks, 2008, page 87).

Wiley Encyclopedia of Forensic Science

In 2009, Wiley InterScience published *The Wiley Encyclopedia of Forensic Science,* described as "the defining major reference work for forensic scientists and the legal profession." This encyclopedia includes an entry on parental alienation syndrome in which the authors said, "This article summarizes parental alienation, a child's rejection of an appropriate parent in the context of a high conflict divorce. Mental health professionals are often asked to evaluate children of separated or divorced parents for the presence of parental alienation. This article explains the psychodynamics and etiology of parental alienation. Custody recommendations and treatment strategies are discussed to aid custody evaluators, judges, and lawyers, and guide families to address this very difficult problem that can destroy families and hurt children" (Kenan and Bernet, 2009).

Ken Lewis, Ph.D.

In 2009, Ken Lewis published a book that was primarily intended for social workers who conduct child custody evaluations, but it is applicable to other mental health professionals. Lewis described a variety of "visitation games" that parents sometimes play, and one was called the "head trip": "The custodial parent repeatedly tells the child that the visitation parent is a bad person in hopes that the child will not want to go on visits. The extreme version of this game may lead to parental alienation whereby the child comes to believe the alienated parent is a bad person and wants to end all visits with that parent. Parental alienation can occur when divorcing parents transform a child into a relationship weapon by engaging in patterns of behavior designed to destroy the child's psychological connection with the other parent" (Lewis, 2009, page 44).

Special Issues of Journals

Numerous mental health practitioners and social researchers have observed parental alienation and published their observations. Hundreds of articles have been published in peer-reviewed mental health and legal journals. (See the comprehensive bibliography on page 187 of this book.) On several occasions, professional journals have devoted special sections or entire issues to parental alienation and related issues of children of divorce.

In 1985, the *Journal of Child Psychiatry* published a special section, "Children of Divorce: Recent Research," which included articles by Hetherington et al. (1985), Wallerstein (1985), and Johnston et al. (1985).

In 2001, the *Family Court Review* published a special issue, "Alienated Children in Divorce." That issue included the important article by Kelly and Johnston (2001), "The Alienated Child: A Reformulation of Parental Alienation Syndrome."

In 2005, the Belgian journal, *Divorce et Séparation* published a special issue, "L'Aliénation Parentale," which included articles by Van

Gijseghem (2005a) and Boch-Galhau and Kodjoe (2005).

Also, in 2005, an Italian journal, *Maltrattamento e Abuso all'Infanzia* devoted a special issue to PAS. That issue included articles by Malagoli Togliatti and Franci (2005) and Malagoli Togliatti and Lubrano Lavadera (2005).

Most recently, in January 2010, the *Family Court Review* published a second special issue regarding parental alienation, which focused on the treatment of this condition. That issue included articles by Warshak (2010a), Sullivan et al. (2010), and Fidler and Bala (2010).

The consistency and redundancy of these publications have confirmed the existence of "a disturbance in which children were preoccupied with deprecation and criticism of a parent—denigration that was unjustified and or exaggerated" (Gardner, 1992a, page 59). Drawing from the numerous collective observations, we consider parental alienation to be a valid concept.

9. Parental alienation is a valid concept. Although it was originally described in the U.S., parental alienation has been identified and studied in many countries.

Parental alienation was originally described in the U.S. independently by six different researchers or research groups, as discussed earlier in this book. Parental alienation has been studied extensively in the U.S., where many mental health and legal professionals have written about it. However, it is extremely important to note that practitioners in many other countries have recognized the same phenomenon. In some cases, these professionals heard about Richard Gardner's criteria for PAS, and they found it helpful to apply those criteria to their own patients and clients. In other cases, the mental health and legal professionals in other countries noticed a particular pattern among the children of high-conflict divorces, and they subsequently realized that these children met the Gardner criteria for PAS. The bibliography of this book cites publications from the professional literature of about 30 countries.

The most exhaustive single volume regarding PAS is *The International Handbook of Parental Alienation Syndrome* (Gardner et al., 2006), which was part of the American Series in Behavioral Science and Law published by Charles C Thomas. More than thirty mental health professionals wrote chapters for this book, including authors from Australia, Canada, the Czech Republic, England, Germany, Israel, Sweden, and the United States. This book received positive reviews. Pressmann (2007) said, "*The International Handbook of Parental Alienation Syndrome* is a powerful volume that provides therapists and justices a wealth of knowledge and wisdom that may positively impact the lives of children who have become fodder in marital and custodial conflicts." Dunkley (2007) said, "The strengths of this volume are its comprehensiveness and its clinical components. There is much to learn from the contributions about how children are manipulated in the aftermath of separation, and how to prevent and repair the damage. I would recommend it to any child welfare professional, particularly those involved in residency and contact disputes."

Argentina

In 1993, the legislature of Argentina adopted a law (Ley 24270) that provides criminal penalties for "a parent or a third person who illegally prevents or obstructs contact of a minor with his or her nonresidential parent." This law has been used to prosecute parents who alienate their children against the other parent. A book by Graciela N. Manonelles, *Responsabilidad penal del padre obstaculizador, La. Ley 24270. Sindrome de alienación parental (SAP) (Criminal Responsibility of the Obstructing Parent, Law 24270. Parental Alienation Syndrome [PAS]),* explains the concept of PAS and also discusses legal cases and prosecution of alienators (Manonelles, 2005).

In 2008, two Argentines, Delia Susana Pedrosa and José Bouza, published an important book, *Síndrome de Alienación Parental. Proceso de obstrucción del vínculo entre los hijos y uno de sus progenitors (Parental Alienation Syndrome: The Process of Obstructing the Bond between the Child and Parent)* (Pedrosa and Bouza, 2008). It is notable that this book received a favorable review in the publication of the National Academy of Sciences of Buenos Aires.

Australia

Sandra S. Berns, Ph.D., a professor at Griffith Law School, Brisbane, has written extensively on family law. She conducted research regarding divorce judgments in Brisbane, Australia, and found that parental alienation syndrome was present in 29 percent of cases (Berns, 2001). In commenting on the role of PAS in family courts in Australia, Berns said, "Although the Australian Family Court will admit evidence of PAS in appropriate cases . . . and has given that evidence weight in decision making, the intense politicization of PAS remains a significant problem for the court. Injudicious statements both by those advocating full legal recognition of PAS and by those opposing such recognition have created a climate in which the courts and the legal profession are skeptical and reluctant to move too far in advance of settled legal and psychiatric opinion" (Berns, 2006).

Belgium

Several mental health professionals in Belgium have observed and written about PAS. A Belgian journal for mental health professionals, *Divorce et Séparation*, devoted its June 2005 issue to the topic of parental alienation. For instance, that issue of the journal included an article by Didier Erwoine, M.A., a Belgian clinical psychologist, "Les traitements du Syndrome d'Aliénation Parentale" ("Treatments of the Parental Alienation Syndrome"). Erwoine said that one of the most dramatic elements of PAS was its often "incurable and irreversible" aspect. In Erwoine's opinion, it is absolutely essential to combine psychotherapeutic treatment with court-ordered measures in order to reverse the PAS inducing process (Erwoine, 2005).

Benoit van Dieren, Ph.D., a psychologist, family therapist, family mediator, and expert, identified PAS in some of the families he assessed in Brussels. He has started to educate mental health and legal professionals regarding this topic. Van Dieren, one of the contributors to this book, reported, "I have always perceived this 'disorder' as a systemic problem, that is, a problem that can be understood only if we consider the complex and dynamic relationships between *at least* three poles: the child, the father, and the mother, plus the other elements gravitating around these poles such as the extended families, friends, new partners, and the judicial and psychosocial systems." In Belgium, van Dieren has helped to organize a multidisciplinary group (a magistrate, a lawyer, a mediator, and a psychologist) to study how to detect PAS and how to intervene when it occurs. They have promoted an approach that is combined (both judicial and psychological functions), coordinated, and rapid.

Jean Yves Hayez, M. D., Ph.D., a child psychiatrist at the Catholic University of Louvain, wrote a cautionary article, "L'Aliénation

Parentale, un concept à haut risque" ("Parental Alienation: A high risk concept") (Hayez and Kinoo, 2005). Hayez thought the concept of parental alienation should be limited to cases in which the toxicity of the guardian parent is evident, for example, in psychotic or highly disturbed parents.

Finally, in 2008, Jean-Emile Vanderheyden, M.D., a neuropsychiatrist, edited and published an important book, *Approcher le divorce conflictuel* (*Approaching the Conflictual Divorce*). This is a multidisciplinary book that discusses high-conflict divorce from a number of perspectives. The chapter authors include judges, lawyers, family mediators, social workers, neuropsychiatrists, and psychologists. The book includes poignant statements by mothers and fathers who experienced loss of their children through parental alienation. There are discussions of the misdiagnosis of parental alienation and the mismanagement of it by the justice system. The authors make various suggestions ranging from the training of competent judges to the designation of "a special day in the calendar" in order to improve societal awareness of parental alienation.

Brazil

Maria Berenice Dias was a distinguished appellate judge who has been a leader in the Brazilian women's movement, particularly fighting against domestic violence. Dias has been active–both in Brazil and internationally–in teaching and writing about family law. Her website (*www.mariaberenicedias.com.br*) includes a notable article, "Síndrome da alienação parental, o que é isso?" ("Parental alienation syndrome, what is it?") (Portuguese). Dias said, "Certainly everyone involved in the study of family conflict and violence in interpersonal relationships has come across a phenomenon that is not new, but that has been identified by more than one name. Some call it 'parental alienation syndrome,' others refer to it as 'implantation of false memories.'" After citing the work of "the American psychiatrist, Richard Gardner," Dias said, "The child, who loves his parent, is taken away from a father who also loves him. This generates a conflict of feelings and a destruction of the bond between them. . . . In this game of manipulation, all weapons are used, including the assertion of the child having been the victim of sexual abuse. . . . The child cannot always discern that he is being manipulated and ends up believing what he was told in such an

insistent and repeated manner. Over time, even the mother cannot distinguish the difference between truth and falsehood. Her truth
becomes the truth for the son, who lives with false characters of a false
existence, resulting then in false memories being implanted in his
mind" (Dias, 2006). Also, Dias edited a book, *Incesto e Alienação
Parental* [*Incest and Parental Alienation*], which contains chapters written
by various professionals involved with family law (Dias, 2007).

Priscilla Maria Pereira Corrêa da Fonseca, Ph.D., a law professor,
published an article in a pediatric journal, "Síndrome de alienação
parental" ("Parental alienation syndrome"). She discussed the causes
of PAS and how to identify it. Corrêa da Fonseca (2006) concluded,
"To identify the parental alienation and prevent this harmful process
from affecting the child and converting into a syndrome are tasks for
the Justice. The family law lawyer must prioritize the child and adolescent even when the alienating parents demand their rights, including the refusal to support the cause of the alienating parent." Igor
Nazarovicz Xaxá wrote a dissertation at Universidade Paulista,
Brasília, which was titled, A Síndrome de Alienação Parental, e o
Poder Judiciário (The Parental Alienation Syndrome and the
Judiciary). Xaxá, who was himself an alienated or targeted parent,
described how Brazilian officials were resistant to appreciating the
serious consequences of PAS (Xaxá, 2008). There is now a proposal in
the National Congress of Brazil to adopt measures (Bill Number
4053/2008) that addresses acts of alienation, seeking to protect children and adolescents from this type of abuse.

Canada

Mental health and legal professionals in Canada have been familiar
with the concept of parental alienation for many years. Perhaps the
earliest discussion of PAS in the professional literature in Canada was
a 1991 article, "Le syndrome d'aliénation parentale," by Anne-France
Goldwater in a law journal (Goldwater, 1991). In 1992, Abe
Worenklein, Ph.D., a clinical and forensic psychologist, published
"Custody Litigation and Parental Alienation." More recently, Gold-
Greenberg and Worenklein (2001) published "L'aliénation Parentale,
un Défi Légal et Clinique pour les Psychologues" ("Parental
Alienation, a Legal and Clinical Challenge for Psychologists").

Hubert Van Gijseghem, Ph.D. (2002, 2004, 2005a, 2009), a professor at the University of Montreal, has conducted research and written extensively regarding parental alienation. For instance, he reported his attempts to calculate the prevalence of parental alienation in metropolitan Montreal in an interesting article, "L'Aliénation parentale: Points controversés" ("Parental alienation: Controversial points"). In that article, Van Gijseghem acknowledged that the concept of parental alienation is not accepted by everybody, and he commented on the emotional debates regarding this topic. He concluded, "That the phenomenon does exist, there is no doubt, but we will have to wait another decade to resolve several aspects of the controversy" (Van Gijseghem, 2005a). Van Gijseghem has also organized training workshops regarding parental alienation for professionals in Canada and European countries.

Marie Hélène Gagné, Ph.D., and Sylvie Drapeau, Ph.D., psychologists at Laval University, Quebec, published "L'aliénation parentale est-elle une forme de maltraitance psychologique?" ("Is parental alienation a form of psychological abuse?"). The authors proposed to use the conceptual and theoretical frame of psychological abuse to study parental alienation. They defined both concepts and described the conceptual links between them (Gagné and Drapeau, 2005).

A progressive Canadian judge, Justice Harvey Brownstone, recently published *Tug of War: A Judge's Verdict on Separation, Custody Battles, and the Bitter Realities of Family Court* (Brownstone, 2009a). In an essay in a major newspaper, Justice Brownstone discussed the differential diagnosis of contact refusal. He said, "Non-custodial parents routinely allege parental alienation when access is denied. The court must first decide if the allegation is valid. Family dynamics are layered and complex, and it is no simple task to find out why a child is refusing to see a noncustodial parent. What is the child's age and stage of development? Does the child have independent reasons stemming from memories of events before the break-up, or relating to the way access is occurring? Has the child been coached, bribed, threatened or manipulated to express negative views about the access parent? Family courts often require the assistance of assessments from psychologists or social workers. This can take time, which intensifies the problem if alienation is occurring" (Brownstone, 2009b).

The Canadian Symposium for Parental Alienation Syndrome (CS-PAS) is an international, educational conference for mental health professionals, family law attorneys and other professionals dedicated to the prevention and treatment of parental alienation and PAS. The CS-PAS conferences occurred in March 2009 and October 2009 in Toronto. Additional information is available at *www.cspas.ca.*

Children Caught in Divorce Battleground
Abe Worenklein, Ph.D., Montreal, Canada

In this case, the parents had two daughters, ages 9 and 11. The mother was extremely distraught when the father informed her that he wanted a divorce because he was not getting the affection he needed in the relationship and because he was tired of the ongoing verbal conflict. Soon thereafter, the father separated from his wife after informing the children he was moving out because he did not want them exposed to the continual conflict.

The father began going out with another woman and, once his wife discovered this, she wanted her daughters to know what was going on. The mother parked her car, with the girls inside, on Friday evenings near the father's home and waited for him to leave the home to go out with his girlfriend. The mother apparently wanted the children to share in her hurt and anger toward the father. Of course, the children became furious at their father when they saw him meeting his girlfriend and they cut off all contact with him and his extended family. They used abusive and vulgar language when they spoke with him and they wanted to have nothing to do with him.

Dr. Worenklein was the jointly mandated expert who evaluated the situation. He noted that the children were ridden with guilt because they blamed themselves for not having done more to keep their parents together. According to Dr. Worenklein, the children refused to see the paternal grandparents and other members of the father's extended family, or to accept phone calls or gifts from them. The children believed that "everybody" knew about their father's new relationship and they avoided getting together with peers. The children felt that they had to be supportive of their mother and to make her feel better.

Dr. Worenklein said that this parental alienation continued for a significant period of time. It started to resolve when the court threatened to change custody from the mother to the father. The court ordered reunification therapy for the children and father together, and also therapy for the mother. The introduction of a new significant other may be the single most common event that hastens parental alienation. Parents need to be aware of this risk when starting a new relationship.

Czech Republic

Eduard Bakalář, C.Sc., is a psychologist who began assessing custody disputes for the Municipal Court in Prague in 1967. He has noted the occurrence of parental alienation in the Czech Republic, where mental health professionals have published articles regarding this topic. Bakalář also reported that the phenomenon of parental alienation has been described in the Ukraine and Russia, but the mental health professionals have no name for it because they are not familiar with the literature and research published elsewhere.

Bakalář wrote extensively regarding parental alienation, including "Popouzení dítete proti druhému rodici" ("Inciting the child against the other parent" (Bakalář and Novák, 1996) and "Syndrom zavrzení rodice: Príciny, diagnóza, terapie" ("Parental alienation syndrome: Etiology, diagnostics, therapy) (Bakalář, 2006b). In his book, *Pruvodce otcovstvím, (A Guide through Fatherhood)*, Bakalář included a chapter regarding parental alienation syndrome in the Czech Republic (Bakalář, 2002). In another book chapter, Bakalář discussed the psychodyamics of PAS. He said, "Competition and narcissism may play a part in the rivalry between some parents who consciously or unconsciously wish that their children will look like, act like, and think like they do. . . . Neurotic egotistical projection on the part of at least one parent can cause the child to favor a point of view and take sides when the child observes parental conflict and separation of the household" (Bakalář, 2006a, page 302).

Denmark

A Danish judge who has written extensively about family law, Svend Danielsen, recently published *Forældres Pligter–Börns Rettigheder (Parents' Duties–Children's Rights)*. This judge was commissioned by Nordisk Ministerrråd (the Nordic Council of Ministers) to compare family law in English-speaking countries (England, Scotland, Australia, and Canada) with the Nordic countries (Denmark, Finland, Iceland, Norway, and Sweden) to look for possible ideas for Nordic reforms. In this book, PAS was mentioned and the phenomenon of parental alienation was discussed: "It can be that the residential parent has such strong rejections against visiting rights for the other parent that the child is affected. In English justice it is called 'implacable hostility.' Another concept and manifestation of conflict is 'parental alienation syndrome.' . . . Generally it is unlucky to capitulate because of ill-disposed parents, resulting in no visitation. . . . If one of the parents makes the contact difficult or impossible, a decision on residence for the child can be altered, but this has to be the last way out, and the possibility cannot be used for solving a relatively mild contact problem" (Danielsen, 2004, pages 210–211).

The Danish organization, Foreningen Far til Støtte for Børn og Forældre (Fathers in Support of Children and Parents) was established in 1977. This organization convened a conference on parental alienation in 2002, and lectures regarding parental alienation and PAS were presented by Erik Kofod and Lena Hellblom Sjögren, Ph.D., a Swedish psychologist. The proceedings of this conference were published in the organization's yearbook, "On Visitation and Parents' Responsibility," in September 2002.

Finland

Anja Hannuniemi, LL.Lic.–a lawyer, licentiate of law, and medical law researcher–has conducted research and taught criminal law and medical law at the University of Helsinki for twenty years. She is preparing a doctor's thesis about PAS. Hannuniemi has acted as an attorney, expert witness, and a judge in very difficult cases involving children. When she heard about PAS in 2000, Hannuniemi immediately realized that PAS had been a factor in all of the longest and most difficult custody disputes and compulsory guardianship cases that she had been working on as an attorney. ("Compulsory guardianship" means that the municipality becomes the custodian of the child instead of the parents.) Hannuniemi thought that in many of these cases, PAS was induced or made much worse by social workers involved with the divorced families. Hannuniemi has worked hard to educate the judiciary in Finland regarding PAS. For instance, in a lengthy article published in a Finnish legal journal, she noted, "Alienation syndrome does not result only from the close parent intentionally, semi-intentionally, or subconsciously acting to alienate the child from the other parent, but its clinical picture also includes *the part of the child,* in which he/she–following his/her sense of loyalty to the close parent–is susceptible to the indoctrination practiced by that parent, and actively alienates oneself from the distant parent" (Hannuniemi, 2007).

France

There is considerable interest in PAS among both mental health professionals and child advocates in France. An advocacy organization, Association Contre l'Aliénation Parentale (ACALPA) (The Association against Parental Alienation) was founded in 2004. This organization engages in extensive education of parents, legal professionals, and mental health professionals regarding PAS. ACALPA also organizes national programs for training police and gendarmerie officers regarding PAS.

French psychiatrists have studied PAS and published papers regarding this topic. Paul Bensussan, M.D., for example, a psychiatric expert for the French courts, has specialized in cases of parental alienation and false allegations of child sexual abuse. In 15 years, he has studied more than 800 cases of high conflict divorce. In a recent article in a medical journal, "L'aliénation parentale: vers la fin du déni?" ("Parental alienation: Toward the end of the denial"), Bensussan commented that PAS "arouses polemics and controversies." He said in the abstract, "Some go as far as denying the very existence of the phenomenon itself, arguing that it is still absent from the international classifications of psychiatric disorders (European or American). . . . The author describes the difficulties encountered, by judges as well as by experts, to evaluate the quality of the relationship before the split and to suggest adequate solutions, in as much as the field of action is severely restricted with such determined children or teenagers" (Bensussan, 2009).

Another psychiatric expert, Jean-Marc Delfieu, M.D., published in a legal journal "Syndrome d'aliénation parentale–Diagnostic et prise en charge médico-juridique" ("Parental alienation syndrome–Diagnosis and medical-legal management"). In that article, Delfieu described the recent increase of cases with severe mental manipulation of children, which he saw in divorce cases. He described the psychopathology, psychodynamics, and clinical manifestation of PAS, with case examples. He proposed joint therapeutic and judicial interventions (Delfieu, 2005).

Mireille Lasbats, Ph.D., a clinical psychologist and forensic expert, published an article in an important legal journal, "Étude du syndrome d'aliénation parentale à partir d'une expertise civile" ("Study of the parental alienation syndrome starting from a civil expertise").

Lasbats described the identification of PAS in high-conflict divorces. With clinical cases she explained how to recognize this phenomenon

---

Infidelity and Parental Alienation
Paul Bensussan, M.D., Versailles, France

In this case, Mr. R and Mrs. R had a difficult marriage and the mother had an affair with another man. The children—Sarah, age 11, and Benjamin, 5—severely reproached the mother for cheating on their father. Mrs. R became destabilized by her children's hostility, and a violent incident occurred. When she was insulted by Sarah, Mrs. R slapped her daughter. Mr. R had to call the police. Mrs. R moved out of the family home.

In the ensuing months, Mrs. R's relationship with her children became worse and worse. Both Sarah and Benjamin became systematically oppositional. Eventually, when Sarah was 12 and Benjamin was 6, the parents definitively separated. After that, the children—united by their hostility against their mother—refused visitation completely and kept repeating, "We want to live with Dad."

The court appointed Dr. Bensussan to evaluate the family. Dr. Bensussan said, "There had been no communication at all—even on the phone—between the children and their mother by the time I was appointed by the judge. The father pretended that he was totally unable to do anything about it. The father said he wanted to re-establish the relationship between the mother and the children, and he admitted his ex-wife had been a good mother." Dr. Bensussan commented that the father appeared to have an enmeshed relationship with the children. He said, "The father seemed to take his children's suffering as his own. Mr. R was ominipresent for his children, hoping that his unfailing affection would compensate for their mother's abandonment." During the course of Dr. Bensussan's evaluation of the family, Mr. R announced that he had been asked to work in the South of France, and he and the children were about to move 800 kilometers from Mrs. R's home.

This vignette illustrates how complex these cases can be. In this family, Sarah and Benjamin had a good excuse to favor their father over their mother. Also, it is understandable that Mr. R became overly solicitous toward the children. However, it was not reasonable for the children to totally reject all contact with their mother. According to Dr. Bensussan, the children's response was greatly out of proportion to anything the mother had done. Furthermore, Mr. R could have done much more to encourage the resumption of contact between Mrs. R and their children.

and the risks to which the alienated child, as well as the rejected parent, are exposed. Consistent with Richard Gardner's concept of PAS, Lasbats said the factors contributing to this condition are the manipulation by a parent and the contribution of the child to the denigration of the rejected parent (Lasbats, 2004).

Also, Jacques Trémintin, M. A., a social worker, published an article, "Quand l'enfant se retrouve piégé–L'aliénation parentale" ("When the child finds himself/herself trapped–Parental alienation") Trémintin said, "The concept of parental alienation seems to be very helpful to better understand what is going on in certain families and work out intervention strategies for professionals" (Trémintin, 2005).

Germany

A large number of German mental health and legal professionals have studied and commented on PAS. The first mention of "Parental Alienation Syndrome (PAS)" in the German professional literature was in 1995 by Wolfgang Klenner, Ph.D., a forensic psychologist, in an important article, "Rituale der Umgangsvereitelung bei getrennt lebenden oder geschiedenen Eltern" ("Rituals of contact refusal from parents in separation or divorce"). Klenner mentioned PAS–when a child has been heavily manipulated by one parent on whom it is dependent–as one of the possible causes of contact refusal (Klenner, 1995).

In 1998, Ursula Kodjoe, M.A. (a forensic psychologist, family therapist, and mediator) and Peter Koeppel, J.D. (a family law attorney) published papers regarding PAS in Germany (Kodjoe and Koeppel, 1998a, 1998b, 1998c). These articles prompted an intensive discussion among mental health and legal professionals in Europe regarding the phenomenon of parental alienation and the diagnosis of parental alienation syndrome. Subsequently, Kodjoe said, "Experts need to have several theories and concepts at their disposal–amongst others, the PAS concept as an explanation for the refusal of contact for *manipulative reasons.* Experts who equate any form of contact refusal and the PAS concept did not understand the concept and must therefore reject it. The 'estranged child' is left out as a consequence. Manipulated against the other by the caretaking parent, seldom by the visiting parent and at the worst by both parents, the child internalizes the enemy image and behaves accordingly. This emotional abuse seems to be a taboo and is denied even by experts" (Kodjoe, 2003b).

Walter Andritzky, Ph.D., a forensic psychologist and sociologist, studied PAS phenomena and published book chapters and articles in professional journals regarding this topic (Andritzky, 2002a, 2002b, 2002c, 2003a, 2003b, 2003c). He published two book chapters regarding PAS in English: Behavioral Patterns and Personality Structure of Alienating Parents: Psychosocial Diagnostic and Orientation Criteria for Intervention (Andritzky, 2003d) and The Role of Medical Reports in the Development of Parental Alienation Syndrome (Andritzky, 2006). Andritzky described the behavioral patterns of alienated children and the personality structure of alienating parents, as well as the "natural" and "induced" symptoms of children affected by high conflict separation or divorce. His articles assist professionals and institutions of the health and legal systems to understand the psychodynamic and diagnostic criteria of PAS and to make appropriate clinical and legal decisions in cases involving PAS.

Wilfrid von Boch-Galhau, M.D., a psychiatrist and psychotherapist, and Ursula Kodjoe studied adult survivors of PAS in Germany. In a book chapter in English, they said, "The induction of PAS in the child must be considered a form of psychological/emotional abuse. It can be connected with traumatizing long-term effects in the child that endure into adulthood. It is difficult to understand that this phenomenon—despite corresponding clinical findings and despite relevant results of recent traumatology and victimology research—is still trivialized, denied, or even opposed by many experts" (Boch-Galhau and Kodjoe, 2006b, page 310). They also published their findings in a French journal, *Synapse, Journal de Psychiatrie et Système Nerveux Central* (Boch-Galhau and Kodjoe, 2006a).

Also, Boch-Galhau, Kodjoe, Koeppel and Andritzky organized the International Conference on PAS that was held in Frankfurt, Germany, in October 2002. Richard Gardner presented a lecture at that conference. The proceedings of this conference were published in their book, *Das Parental Alienation Syndrom: Eine interdisziplinäre Herausforderung für scheidungsbegleitende Berufe (The Parental Alienation Syndrome: An Interdisciplinary Challenge for Professionals Involved with Divorce)* (Boch-Galhau et al., 2003). Information regarding this conference can be found on *www.pas-konferenz.de*.

Astrid Camps, M.D., a child psychiatrist in Germany, said, "Gardner's PAS concept proves helpful in child psychiatric practice. If the PAS problem for the child of divorce is not solved, the psychiatric

Father Excludes Mother from Their Children's Lives
Wilfrid von Boch-Galhau, M.D., Würzburg, Germany

Dr. Boch-Galhau has studied targeted parents and adult children of parental alienation. For example, he interviewed a woman, Mrs. D, who left an abusive husband and her children, a 16-year-old son and 13-year-old daughter.

For about a year, Mrs. D had regular contact with her children, but then noticed that they were distancing themselves from her. Mrs. D's son sent her this message: "If you don't return to the side of your husband, you'll never see me again." The son carried out this threat, and he refused to see his mother again to this day.

Then, the father gave Mrs. D's daughter the following choice: "You either join your mother, then you will never see us again. Or, you stay with us, then you will not see your mother anymore." Later, the girl's father and brother gave her the following choice on December 23: "Either you stay here on Christmas Eve or you never see us again." Three years later, the daughter, age 16, escaped from the father's house in order to live with her mother. As a consequence, her father and brother broke off all contact with her to this day.

Over time, Mrs. D met other women in Germany with similar experiences. In the interview with Dr. Boch-Galhau, Mrs. D poignantly said, "There are more and more affected women. This is becoming apparent. To deal with it is infinitely painful and difficult. It is not only that one has lost the children, also the time is irretrievable. . . . One also has one's feelings as a mother, which are amputated from one day to the next. It is not possible to carry on. Where to put the emotions, the mothering in which one was just engulfed?"

Of course, Mrs. D became involved with attorneys, judges, the youth welfare authority, a guardian *ad litem,* and a psychologist. She learned about parental alienation and PAS on the Internet. At the conclusion of the interview, Mrs. D said, "It would have been helpful if my attorney had known anything about PAS. Just as important it would have been if my therapist had known anything about it. . . . The youth welfare office . . . felt unable to deal with the situation. I had the feeling they were at the end of their options, they no longer had means to really intervene, and they also shied away from the necessary decision."

More information about this family and similar cases involving adults affected by parental alienation may be found in the book chapter by Boch-Galhau and Kodjoe (2006b).

and psychosomatic long-term consequences can be dramatic and for the child patient may be accompanied by great suffering (Camps, 2003, page 155).

Uwe Jopt, Ph.D., and Katharina Behrend, Ph.D., forensic psychologists from the University of Bielefeld, published a well-known pair of articles regarding PAS. They described PAS as consisting of two stages. In the first stage, the specific conditions for the development of PAS are met (instrumentalization and parentification of the child, denigration of the other parent, with the custodial parent expecting the child to align to herself). In the second stage, the syndrome is solidified. There occurs a reduction of cognitive dissonance, a lack of empathy, internal and external reinforcement. The authors discussed possible methods of intervention by the various professions (family court, social services, psychological experts, and lawyers) (Jopt and Behrend, 2000a, 2000b).

In Germany, mental health and legal professionals, institutions, and agencies use an important handbook, *Kindesmisshandlung und Vernachlässigung (Child Abuse and Neglect)*. This book refers to the "Parental Alienation Syndrome" as a particular kind of psychological violence against children in the context of custody and visitation conflicts (Deegener and Körner, 2005, pages 684 and 694).

Israel

Daniel J. Gottleib, Psy.D., is a clinical psychologist who has served as a court appointed expert in child custody and adoption cases. In a book chapter, Gottleib said, "In the Hebrew literature, PAS is referred to by different names: syndrome *nikur hori* (parental alienation syndrome), *hitnakrut he-horeh* (alienation from a parent), or *sarvanut kesher* (contact refusal). The differences in terminology do not reflect different theoretical approaches, . . . but rather all point to the same constellations of symptoms and dynamics that comprise PAS as described by Gardner" (Gottleib, 2006, page 90).

Italy

Several mental health professionals in Italy have published articles, book chapters, and books regarding parental alienation. Apparently, the first person to write about PAS in the Italian professional literature was Isabella Buzzi, Ph.D., who is on the faculty of the Catholic University of Milan. Buzzi contributed a chapter regarding PAS to a comprehensive book, *Separazione, Divorzio e Affidamento dei Figli (Separation, Divorce, and Child Custody)* (Buzzi, 1997). In the following year, Guglielmo Gulotta published "La sindrome di alienazione genitoriale: Definizione e descrizione" ("The parental alienation syndrome: Definition and description") (Gulotta, 1998).

A psychologist, Roberto Giorgi, has written extensively regarding parental alienation, including a monograph, *Le Possibili Insidie delle Child Custody Disputes: Introduzione Critica alla Sindrome di Alienazione Parentale di Richard A. Gardner (The Possible Pitfalls of Child Custody Disputes: Critical Introduction to Parental Alienation Syndrome by Richard A. Gardner)* (Giorgi, 2005). Mario Andrea Salluzzo, a psychologist and psychotherapist, reviewed and summarized the work of Richard Gardner regarding PAS, and applied the concepts to several Italian cases. In a journal article, Salluzzo concluded, "For a therapeutic intervention, it is necessary that the legal personnel and the mental health professionals work in synergy. Only a clear and swift judicial action, aimed to discourage any attempt of sabotage by the alienating parent, can guarantee a good margin of success for psychotherapeutic or family mediation interventions" (Salluzzo, 2006).

In 2005, an entire issue of a professional journal, *Maltrattamento e Abuso all'Infanzia (Maltreatment and Abuse of Children)* was devoted to PAS. The articles included "La sindrome di alienazione genitoriale (PAS): Studi e ricerche" ("The parental alienation syndrome (PAS): Studies and research") (Malagoli Togliatti and Franci, 2005) and "La sindrome di alienazione genitoriale (PAS): Epigenesi relazionali" ("The parental alienation syndrome (PAS): Epigenesis of relationships") (Malagoli Togliatti and Lubrano Lavadera, 2005). Marisa Malagoli Togliatti is a professor for the psychodynamics of child development and family relations at a distinguished institution, Sapienza Università di Roma.

There is a comprehensive, recent book from Italy regarding parental alienation, *La Sindrome di Alienazione Parentale (PAS): Lavaggio del Cervello e Programmazione dei Figli in Danno Dell'altro Genitore (The Parental Alienation Syndrome [PAS]: Brainwashing and Programming of Children to the Detriment of the Other Parent).* The authors include: Guglielmo Gulotta, a psychologist, lawyer, and professor of forensic psychology at the University of Turin; Adele Cavedon, a researcher in the Department of Psychology at the University of Padua; and Moira Liberatore, a psychologist, mediator, and lecturer at the University of Turin. They provide a complete and systematic description of PAS and its manifestations, generally based on the work of Richard Gardner, with a discussion of the differential diagnosis of PAS and related topics such as false memories and factitious disorder by proxy. These authors developed a method for identifying alienating behavior by means of microanalysis of communicative interaction and psycholinguistic analysis. This method involved the careful study of dialogue between the alienating parent and the child. They intended "to provide the various professional groups who encounter this perverse condition precise directions to recognize, diagnose, denounce, and take charge" (Gulotta et al., 2008).

The concept of parental alienation has been recognized by the mental health and legal communities in Italy. Professor Gulotta, one of the contributors to this book, reported that the Italian Parliament has recently considered two bills regarding shared custody "because of the need to put an end to the attempt by one parent to completely oust the other parent." The proposals for these bills refer specifically to PAS. Also, trial courts sometimes refer to "parental alienation" and "parental alienation syndrome" in their decisions.

Japan

Colin P. A. Jones, a professor at Doshisha Law School, Kyoto, Japan, discussed parental alienation in an article, "In the Best Interests of the Court: What American Lawyers Need to Know about Child Custody and Visitation in Japan." He said, "Unfortunately, focusing on the problem as a cross-cultural one risks marginalizing it. In reality, parental child abduction and parental alienation are problems for parents and children in Japan, regardless of race or nationality. For every foreign parent who loses contact with their children in Japan, a greater number of Japanese parents suffer the same fate" (Jones, 2007).

Malaysia

In conducting this research, we found very little information regarding the occurrence and recognition of parental alienation in Islamic countries. However, we did locate an essay, "When Fathers Move Out of the Home," that was written by a professor at the law school of the International Islamic University Malaysia, Dr. Zaleha Kamarudin, LL.B., Ph.D. Dr. Kamarudin is an expert in Islamic law and has written or edited fourteen books regarding Malaysian family law and related issues. In her essay, Dr. Kamarudin discussed the various reasons why fathers become less involved and excluded from their children's lives. She said, "Children are often drawn into conflict between parents and are forced to take sides, which are not only stressful but result in a deterioration in father-child relationships. . . . Parental alienation syndrome has been confirmed by many studies to be the main reason for the lack of contact. Many noncustodial fathers interviewed in that study believed that their former wives were poisoning the children's mind against them, or they were blocking their access to the children by making physical or telephone contact difficult" (Kamarudin, 2009).

Mexico

The First International Congress of Families was held in Mexico City in August 2006. The congress participants passed resolutions including the following: "It is important to stress that children should not suffer the consequences of separation or divorce of the parents. . . . Manipulating the children to create hatred or bitterness toward any of the parents, that is, parental alienation, should be avoided." It was noted that the manipulation and brainwashing of children should be considered a form of child abuse. An international congress specifically regarding "Síndrome de Alienación Parental" took place in June 2009 in Monterey, Mexico.

Apparently, the legislature of the state of Querétaro, Mexico, has been particularly proactive in recognizing the issue of parental alienation among divorced parents. The recently revised Civil Code of Querétaro states in Article 396, "Whosoever exercises parental authority over a dependent minor ought to procure the establishment of a respectful and close relationship between said minor and the other adult exercising parental authority over this minor. Each adult exercising such parental authority over the minor must avoid any act of manipulation or parental alienation that may lead to feelings of resentment or rejection by said minor for the other adult" (Instituto de Investigaciones Jurícas, 2009).

The Netherlands

Ed Spruijt, Ph.D., at Utrecht University and his colleagues conducted quantitative research regarding PAS. They sent questionnaires to members of the Dutch Association of Family Lawyers and Divorce Mediators and also to a group of nonresident parents. Altogether they had 138 respondents from these two groups, and the authors "aimed to gain a first empirical impression of the phenomena of PAS in the Netherlands." In conclusion, the authors stated, "Does parental alienation occur in the Netherlands? Our research confirms that it does. Of the respondents to our questionnaire, 58% thought PAS does not occur, or hardly, in the Netherlands, whereas 42% thought it does occur" (Spruijt et al., 2005).

Norway

In 1994, Richard Gardner introduced the concept of PAS to Norway when he spoke at a conference called "Seksuelle overgrep mot barn rettssikkerhet og rasjonalitet" ("Child Sexual Abuse, Justice and Rationality"). Part of Gardner's lecture was later published in a book, *Seksuelle overgrep mot barn: Et kritisk perspektiv (Child Sexual Abuse: A Critical Perspective),* which was edited by Astrid Holgerson, Ph.D., and Hellblom Sjögren, Ph.D. (1997). Probably the first description of parental alienation by a professional in Norway was an article by Jan Brögger, an anthropologist, who wrote, "Når barn utvikler sykelig hat mot foreldre" ("When Children Develop Morbid Hatred toward Parents") (Brögger, 1995).

A psychiatrist in Oslo, Terje Torgersen, M.D., has published several newspaper articles regarding parental alienation. In an article called "Foreldrehat-syndromet" ("Parental Hate Syndrome"), he wrote, "If a residence parent frightens the child to reject contact with the other parent although he/she has visiting rights, this strategy will often be successful. As long as our politicians do not realize how serious the situation is, there is little hope for changes of the law (sole custody is still the norm)" (Torgersen, 1995b). In an article called "Samvaersrett og avmakt" ("Visitation Rights and Powerlessness"), Torgersen commented on the pathology often found in alienating parents. He wrote, "A lot of parents, sabotaging their children's legitimate contact with the other parent, sadly enough have more or less disturbed personalities and are not capable of focusing on their children's needs instead of their own. It is noteworthy that the society has not done more to help these children by reassuring them an actual right to have contact with both their parents" (Torgersen, 2008b).

There have been additional publications in Norway regarding parental alienation and closely related topics. A Norwegian professor of psychology, Frode Thuen, published a book regarding children of divorced parents, *Livet Som Deltidsforeldre (Life as a Part-time Parent)*. One of the chapters describes programming of a child to reject a parent without justified cause in connection with PAS (Thuen, 2004, pages 91–121). Another important recent book was published by a Norwegian lawyer, Sverre Kvilhaug, a specialist in family law. This book, which discusses research regarding children separated from parents, was *Atskillelse barn og foreldre, Hva internasjonal forskning sier om sammenheng mellom atskillelse I barndommen og senere fysiske og psykiske lidelser (Separation of Children and Parents: What International Research Says about the Relationship between Childhood Separation and Later Physical and Mental Disorders)* (Kvilhaug, 2005). Finally, a Norwegian journalist, Ole Texmo, wrote a pamphlet on how to distinguish mild from serious parental alienation, which was based on a U.S. publication: *Et langt og vanskelig ord Om metodisk påvisning av olike typer av foreldrefiendtliggjöring med referanse til Bone & Walsh (1999) kriterier for identifisering av PAS (Parental Alienation Syndrome (A Long and Difficult Word: The Methodically Detection of Different Types of Parental Alienation with Reference to the Bone & Walsh (1999) Criteria for the Identification of PAS [Parental Alienation Syndrome])* (Texmo, 2007).

Poland

PAS has been observed in Poland and studied by senior academic psychiatrists. In Poland, PAS is called "Zespół Gardnera" or "Gardner Syndrome." For example, Irena Namyslowska, M.D., Ph.D., the head of the Department of Child Psychiatry at the Institute of Psychiatry and Neurology, Warsaw, and her colleagues recently published an article in *Psychiatria Polska*. The title of the article was "Zespół Gardnera–zespół oddzielenia od drugoplanowego opiekuna (PAS). Rozpoznanie czy rzeczywistość rodzinna?" ("Gardner Syndrome–Parent Alienation Syndrome (PAS). Diagnosis or family reality?"). These authors discussed the features of PAS as described by Gardner, and they made suggestions for differentiating that syndrome from actual psychological, physical, and sexual abuse. They said that the symptoms typically seen in parental alienation (the eight behaviors described by Gardner) are different than the symptoms typically seen in physically or sexually abused children (e.g., symptoms of posttraumatic stress disorder). The consequences of "Gardner Syndrome" for legal decisions in court cases involving child custody and the critique of this syndrome in forensic and psychiatric literature are also discussed, and several questions posed. These authors conceptualized PAS not as a disorder of the child, but as "a specific, dynamic family situation, which sometimes occurs during divorce and fights over child custody" (Namyslowska et al., 2009).

A psychologist in Poland–Monika Dreger–also summarized the work of Richard Gardner. Dreger said, in effect, "[Gardner] described a disorder occurring in children, which in the course of the conflict, is involved in deprecation and criticism of one of the parents, but this kind of vilification is not justified and/or exaggerated. PAS can apply only if the children rejected a parent who is not the perpetrator of sexual, physical, or mental abuse against the children." She concluded, "The most important thing is not to involve the child in conflict with the former partner" (Dreger, 2007).

Portugal

Instituto Português Mediação Familiar (the Portuguese Institute for Family Mediation) has produced a pamphlet called "Síndrome de Alienaçào Parental: Abuso psicológico e mau trato infantile!" (Parental Alienation Syndrome: Psychological Abuse and Child Maltreatment." This pamphlet contains a detailed checklist for how to recognize parental alienation.

A Spanish psychologist, José Manuel Aguilar, Ph.D., published a book about PAS in Portuguese, *Síndrome de Alienaçào Parental* (Aguilar, 2008b). Subsequently, Aguilar lectured on this topic at the School of the Judiciary and Bar in Lisbon and other locations in Portugal.

South Africa

Christopher P. Szabo, Ph.D., at the University of the Witwatersrand, Johannesburg, South Africa, has written extensively about psychology and psychiatry in his country. He studied the concept of PAS as it occurred in South Africa. Szabo commented, "Involvement of mental health professionals who have no insight into PAS may exacerbate matters. The longer the time spent with the alienating parent, the more likely the process of alienation will be consolidated. It is suggested that PAS be recognized as a form of child abuse; accordingly custody may be awarded to the innocent party, with sanctions potentially applied against the alienating party" (Szabo, 2002).

Spain

Parental alienation has been recognized and studied extensively in Spain. Probably the most prolific author and speaker regarding parental alienation has been José Manuel Aguilar, Ph.D., a forensic psychologist. Aguilar (2004) published a book regarding this topic, *S.A.P., Síndrome de Alienación Parental.* He also published "Interferencias de las relaciones paterno filiales. El Síndrome de Alienación Parental y las nuevas formas de violencia contra la infancia" ("Interference of the Parent-Child Relationships. Parental Alienation Syndrome and New Forms of Violence against Children") (Aguilar, 2007). Aguilar has lectured at scholarly meetings and at government agencies throughout Spain, as well as in Mexico and Portugal. Aguilar reported that he has documented hundreds of cases of PAS.

Domènec Luengo Ballester, Ph.D., a psychotherapist, and Arantxa Coca Vila, an educational psychologist, have published two books regarding parental alienation. Their first book–*Hijos manipulados tras la separación: Cómo detectar y tratar la alienación parental (Children Manipulated after Separation: How to Detect and Treat Parental Alienation)*–illustrated and explained the messages that parents use to program their children (Luengo Ballester and Coca Vila, 2007). Their second book, recently published–*El sindrome de alienación parental: 80 preguntas y respuestas (The Parental Alienation Syndrome: 80 Questions and Answers)*–explained the difference between parental alienation and loyalty conflicts in children (Luengo Ballester and Coca Vila, 2009).

Mercé Cartié and her colleagues assigned to the Catalan Civil Family Courts conducted research regarding the occurrence of PAS, as defined by Richard Gardner, in the families that came to their attention. They identified 83 children in 69 families who manifested PAS, which constituted about 10 percent in the total population served. These researchers found that over time some children developed false memories of past events. They also found that the various symptoms of PAS occurred with different frequencies in children of different ages (Cartié et al., 2005).

Asunción Tejedor Huerta, Ph.D., who has taught courses for the Official College of Psychologists in Spain, published a book, *El Síndrome de alienación Parental. Una forma de maltrato (Parental Alienation Syndrome. A Form of Abuse)* (Tejedor Huerta, 2007a), as well as articles and book chapters. For example: "Intervención ante el Síndrome de Alienación Parental" ("Response to the Parental Alienation Syndrome") (Tejedor Huerta, 2007b); "SAP y Maltrato" ("PAS, a Form of Abuse") (Tejedor Huerta, 2008); "Pautas de Intervención ante casos de SAP en la familia" ("Intervention in Cases of Parental Alienation Syndrome") (Tejedor Huerta, 2009); and "Reflexiones sobre el Síndrome de Alienación Parental" ("Reflections about the Parental Alienation Syndrome") (Tejedor Huerta, 2006).

Several other Spanish psychologists have written articles regarding parental alienation. Bolaños (2002) published "El síndrome de alienación parental. Descripción y abordajes psico-legales" ("The parental alienation syndrome. Description and psycho-legal approaches"). Gómez (2008) published "Síndrome de Alienación Parental (SAP)." Ramirez (2004) published "Psicología y derecho de familia. Trastorno mental y alternativa de custodia. El síndrome de alienación parental" ("Psychology and family law. Mental disorder and alternative care. Parental Alienation Syndrome").

Adolfo Jarne Esparcia and Mila Arch Marin (2009) considered whether PAS should be included in DSM-5, and they concluded that it should be considered a relational problem. These authors eloquently stated, "In this section [of the DSM] there is a subsection denominated 'relational problems.' . . . It seems evident from the descriptive perspective PAS includes a pattern of interaction of a relational unit (parents and children), which results in a clinically significant impairment in functioning (marked presence of psychological pain and risk in the psychosocial development of the minor given the complete absence of one of the parents) and it can appear related to a pathology in one or more of the unit members or in the absence of any other disorder. And, of course, they are subject to receiving clinical attention; thus, it does not seem that there is any clinician in the world that when confronted with a child who 'does not want to see his/her parent, does not want to have any sort of relationship with him/her' will deal with it with a simple 'that is not important, let him/her not see him/her; it will pass.' This simply does not happen."

Several professional organizations or agencies in Spain have commented on the importance of parental alienation. In 2005, the Ethics Committee of the Official College of Physicians of Madrid denounced the "emotional abuse of children by using them as weapons, as achieved through programming and brainwashing . . . this process is child abuse . . . you get to express a hatred of the minor toward the target parent." In 2007, the Spanish Ministry of Labor and Immigration presented a course regarding PAS for professionals. The objectives of this course were: "Analyze and study the manifestations and consequences of Parental Alienation Syndrome (PAS). Provide skills for the development of competent diagnoses in cases of PAS and planning for more successful intervention in each case. Explore ways of competent intervention in cases where these situations occur." Also, in 2008, the General College of Psychologists in Spain released a statement in which the Coalition of Legal Psychology endorsed "the appropriateness of the analysis of the problem known as Parental Alienation Syndrome in the psychological evaluation . . . within the forensic field of family law." Courts in Spain have endorsed the concept of parental alienation as a factor that they should take into consideration in divorce proceedings.

At least four national and international conferences have been organized in Spain regarding parental alienation. In March 2006, the First National Symposium on Parental Alienation Syndrome took place in Madrid. The participants of that meeting–physicians, psychologists, and attorneys–signed a declaration to the effect, "The manipulation of children by one of the parents, or within the family circle of this parent, with the intention that they reject the other parent, is a type of psychological violence which qualifies as child abuse. This abuse process includes obstruction of the relationship between the children, their parent, and the parent's side of the extended family, false accusations of sexual aggression and abuse, physical distancing mechanisms and inculcation of denigrating and injurious arguments which construct in the mind of the child beliefs, emotions and behaviors which the children believe they themselves have created, in which they express hated against the rejected parent, together with an extreme form of defense of the alienating parent." In December 2008, a second national conference that addressed parental alienation took place in Santiago de Compostela, Galicia, Spain. An international congress, "Síndrome de Alienación Parental y Custodia Compartida," occurred in September 2009, in Léon, Spain. A second international congress occurred in May 2010 in Madrid. (See *www.congresointerna cionalsap.org* for additional information.)

Sweden

The phenomenon of parental alienation in high-conflict custody cases has been described in Sweden. Legal professionals, social workers, and psychologists in Sweden have observed, lectured about, and written about PAS. In 1991, Richard Gardner lectured in Lund, Sweden, on PAS and how to differentiate accurate accusations of child abuse from false accusations often appearing in complex custody conflicts.

In 1992, an important research project was published in Sweden, which was based on interviews with children who had grown up without their fathers. PAS was described in a book, *Pappa, se mig! Om förnekade barn och maktlösa fader, (Father, See Me! About Rejected Children and Powerless Fathers)*. In that book, the researchers related what the children told about their feeling of loss. One child explained her longing to be allowed to love both her parents by saying, "Both are in my blood circulation" (Öberg and Öberg, 1992, page 147).

A Swedish psychologist, Lena Hellblom Sjögren, Ph.D., has extensively studied PAS. In 1997, Hellblom Sjögren described PAS in a book about research on memory, suggestibility, and four criminal cases involving sexual abuse. This book was *Hemligheter och minnen. Att utreda tillförlitlighet i sexualbrottmål (Secrets and Memories: To Investigate Reliability in Sexual Criminal Cases)*. Hellblom Sjögren has practiced as an investigative psychologist giving testimony about PAS in family and criminal courts in Sweden and Norway since the beginning of the 1990s. In several cases, in which Hellblom Sjögren conducted investigations and identified PAS, the court gave custody to the parent who demonstrated insight regarding the importance for the children to have contact with both of their parents. Also, Hellblom Sjögren is a researcher, who is now analyzing how children's human rights and their best interests were affected in 60 cases in which she identified

PAS. Hellblom Sjögren reported cases in which the PAS was brought about by child welfare workers. In a book chapter, Hellblom Sjögren wrote, "The purpose of this article is to describe the alienation process in five Swedish cases where children have developed PAS after having been influenced to reject their mothers by local social welfare agencies. It is concluded that children and their parents are best served if PAS can be recognized, and efforts made to educate professionals about how harmful it can be" (Hellblom Sjögren, 2006, page 131).

In 1998, a child advocacy organization, Rädda Barnen (Save the Children) in Sweden, published an important book, *Barnets rätt till båda föräldrarna (The Child's Right to Both Parents)*. In this book, a Swedish child psychiatrist, Magnus Kihlbom, M.D., wrote about the PAS phenomenon without actually naming it. In a chapter called "Relationen till föräldrarna–grunden för barnets psykiska utveckling" ("The Relation to the Parents–The Foundation for the Child's Mental Development"), Kihlbom said, "It is particularly difficult for a child when a parent's demand for loyalty is so total that it also includes the way to value the other parent. Then the child is threatened to be in disgrace and rejected: if you do not think as I do, if you do not reject him/her, I will reject you in the same way. Many children live in such a situation full of pain, without being able to afford emotionally to protest" (Kihlbom, 1998, page 16).

In 2005, two social workers in Sweden, Gösta Emtestam and Agnetha Svensson, published a book in which they described a method for rapidly investigating the possibility of PAS and then intervening so that alienation resulting in PAS can be avoided. Their goal is for the child to have access to both parents after the parents' separation. The book was *Vårdnads-, boende- och umgängesutredningar (Custody-, Residence- and Visitation-investigations)* (Emtestam and Svensson, 2005).

False Allegations and Parental Alienation
Lena Hellblom Sjögren, Ph.D., Fagersta, Sweden

Dr. Hellblom Sjögren has investigated many cases in which social service personnel and examining physicians have contributed

continued on next page

to the creation of false allegations and parental alienation. In this case, the parents separated in the early 1990s. The two daughters were Eva, age 4, and Lena, age 2. Several weeks later, the mother consulted a child psychiatrist and said: the father was mentally ill (which was not true); Eva had recurrent genital infections (which was not true); and that the father had sexually abused both Eva and Lena (which was later proved to be untrue). However, the child psychiatrist took the mother's statements at face value and wrote in her notes: "The most important thing for the moment is that the children are protected from their biological father. As he is mentally ill, he should not have charge of the children at all as far as I can see."

The psychiatrist's colleague, a child psychologist, interviewed the girls. Although the girls denied that they had been sexually abused, the psychologist said: "The fact that Eva doesn't tell me about sexual abuse is not something that disproves she has been sexually abused. Rather, it suggests the opposite." The psychologist based her opinion—that the children had been sexually abused—on what the children had allegedly told their mother.

The police investigators, who questioned the girls, assumed the girls had been sexually abused based on the history provided by the mother. One of the police interviewers asked leading questions such as: "And Daddy's willy, where was it on you?" "Was your Daddy's willy on your private place?" "Point, Eva, where was your Daddy's willy?"

Ultimately, after an independent investigation by Dr. Hellblom Sjögren, the father was found not guilty of sexually abusing Eva and Lena. However, the children were not allowed to see their father because their mother said they feared him. Subsequently, the court appointed another child psychiatrist to evaluate the children and make recommendations regarding their contact with their father. The child psychiatrist said: "The children developed such a fear of their father that their facial expressions and words demonstrate discomfort and hatred at every mention of him. They became extremely panicked in situations that might result in their having any form of contact with him." Although he doubted that sexual abused had occurred, he concluded that Eva and Lena should be protected "against a potential risk of abuse."

Seventeen years later, Eva and Lena have not seen their father. Dr. Hellblom Sjögren commented: "The phrase to best describe what has happened is 'authority abuse.' Bearing in mind the traditionally accepted division of power, social workers have totally incompatible tasks: they investigate, they make decisions, they execute these decisions, and they evaluate their own decisions and actions."

Switzerland

Mental health and legal professionals in Switzerland have observed and written about PAS. For example, Ursula Birchler-Hoop, a Swiss family law attorney and mediator, published "Eltern-Entfremdung, Störungen im Kontakt zwischen dem Kind und dem nicht-sorge-berechtigten Elternteil" ("Parent-child alienation, contact difficulties between child and noncustodial parent") (German). Birchler-Hoop provided a detailed discussion of the symptoms, diagnosis, causes, and psychodynamics of the parental alienation syndrome, as well as possible methods of intervention. Regarding PAS and Swiss family law practice, Birchler-Hoop noted that from the legal literature and case law one can conclude that there is general awareness of the problem of parent-child alienation in Switzerland, but solid knowledge about PAS is still mostly lacking (Birchler-Hoop, 2002).

Also, Pedro Goncalves, M. D., a psychiatrist and family therapist, and A. Grimaud de Vincenzi, a family consultant, published an article, "D'ennemis à Coéquipiers, le Difficile Apprentissage de la Coparentalité après un Divorce Conflictuel" ("Co-parenting after a conflicted divorce, growing from enemy to ally") (French). The authors said that in the process of a conflictual divorce, the children are almost always caught in the triangle of their parents' fights. Their description of the process corresponded with Richard Gardner's description of the parental alienation syndrome. The authors explained intervention techniques aimed at de-triangulating the children and helping the parents achieve collaboration as a functional parenting team. The authors stressed potential traps and the need to coordinate therapeutic interventions with the courts involved in the custody decisions (Goncalves and Vincenzi, 2003).

United Kingdom

Several English mental health professionals have studied, described, and commented on parental alienation. Ludwig F. Lowenstein, Ph.D., has been a practicing psychologist in England for over 40 years. A prolific author, he has published over 400 articles and a dozen books, including articles and book chapters regarding PAS (e.g., Lowenstein, 1998, 2006a, 2006c). Lowenstein's book, *Parental Alienation Syndrome: How to Understand and Address Parental Alienation Resulting from*

Acrimonious Divorce or Separation, was published in 2007. Lowenstein addressed in detail the causes of parental alienation and possible treatment approaches. For example, he said, "The inducer of the implacable hatred holds the key to the child's delusional beliefs of the absent parent. If this parent (with or without counseling) learns to self-reflect and stimulate the child in their relationship with the other parent, then the child's delusional beliefs of the absent parent and their 'evil and wicked ways' can be eliminated. Often this is not the case and the custodial parent persists in promoting rejection of the absent parent in the child. Only by breaking the relationship between the inducer of such implacable hatred towards the absent parent can the child's delusional beliefs be eliminated" (Lowenstein, 2007, page 47).

Kirk Weir, M.D., a child, adolescent, and family psychiatrist, has observed and described parental alienation. In a journal article, Weir (2006) listed the eight characteristics of PAS including the campaign of denigration and the weak, absurd, or frivolous rationalizations for the denigration. Weir said, "The phenomena . . . have been witnessed by the author in scores of cases, and in their most extreme manifestation the effect was to create a sense of *fear and/or loathing of one parent*–the child may state that they are terrified at the prospect of any contact, and may give this appearance" (Weir, 2006).

Tony Hobbs, J.P., L.L.M., a psychologist and researcher in family law, teaches at Keele University, England. In a book chapter, Hobbs said, "As PAS becomes more widely accepted, undoubtedly instances will arise in which false and/or malicious claims of children being inculcated into PAS are made. This may be regrettable but it should not be surprising, as it will only represent the converse of the many false claims of abuse that have become prevalent against PAS target parents" (Hobbs, 2006b, page 89).

Dr. Celest L. van Rooyen (a clinical psychologist) and Dr. Bala Mahendra (a psychiatrist and a lawyer) recently published *Psychology in Family and Child Law.* In the chapter on "Parental Alienation," they said, "Parental Alienation Syndrome is a pervasive social problem with far-reaching and potentially permanent repercussions for the child. When alienation becomes complete, it can amount to a complete termination of parental rights, the alienated child having experienced the loss of nuclear and extended family, in addition to other long-term, detrimental effects (van Rooyen and Mahendra, 2007).

10. Parental alienation is a valid concept. Collateral research regarding related topics supports the contention that parental alienation is a real phenomenon.

Several strands of research and theory—outside of that specifically devoted to children of divorce—are consistent with the existence of parental alienation as a genuine phenomenon. These lines of research and theory relate to the etiology of parental alienation, its manifestation, and its maintenance in troubled families. Areas of interest include the following: psychoanalysis; cognitive dissonance theory; research regarding false beliefs and false memories; research regarding parental loss; national and international protocols regarding the rights of children; emotional abuse of children; domestic violence; the competency of children to testify; family systems theory; and psycholinguistic analysis.

Psychoanalysis

While psychodynamic scholarship typically deals with the intrapsychic experience of individuals, some authors have studied the preconscious and unconscious substrate of relationships that involve two or more individuals. David M. Levy, M.D., for instance, conducted extensive research on maternal overprotection in the 1930s. He and his colleagues searched through more than 2,000 cases at the Institute for Child Guidance in New York City, from which they selected twenty cases of maternal overprotection "in its simplest and clearest form." Although Levy had never heard of "parental alienation," he described all the components of that phenomenon in his book, *Maternal Overprotection,* Levy said, "Take the case of a mother who soon after the birth of her child manifests a strong overprotective attitude. She 'lives only for her child.' Her life is devoted to him. She is uncomfortable whenever she is away from him, if only for a few minutes. She allows the husband to have little or no share in her baby's training. It is her baby, not his. She threatens to leave the house if her husband dare lay a finger to the child. The husband's role as father is negligible and remains so throughout the life of the child" (Levy, 1943, page 16). Levy then described the fathers of these children: "These fathers appear . . . readily adaptable to such compete surrender of the paternal role by virtue of their generally submissive traits" (Levy, 1943, page 151). Also, he described the children themselves: "To these facts must be added the derogatory attitude of the child toward the father, which is in some instances fostered by the mother, thereby reducing the paternal influence to its lowest degree" (Levy, 1943, page 153).

An extreme form of parental overprotection may take the form of *folie à deux.* Two psychoanalysts, E. James Anthony, M.D., and Therese Benedek, M.D., described *folie à deux* in the following manner: "These mothers consciously induce and deliberately maintain the emotional symbiosis far beyond the psychophysiogic needs of the children. . . . Fostering a strong dependency on themselves, they isolate their children from other children and from adults. The unconscious communication is maintained through the transactional processes of the manifest and often goal-conscious behavior of the mothers whose reactions sharpen the children's anticipation so that they gradually become automatons, surrendering their volition to the mothers who remain, despite all their pathologic conditions, surrogate egos" (Anthony and Benedek, 1970, page 572).

After parental alienation was recognized and named, several authors noted that some severe cases of parental alienation resemble *folie à deux.* For example, Elizabeth M. Ellis, Ph.D., said, "Both Richard Gardner and Janet Johnston mention the similarity between severely alienated or aligned children and the phenomenon of *folie à deux.* . . . A brief review of what is known about *folie à deux* reveals striking similarities to PAS. Essentially, the core feature of *folie à deux* is that a delusion develops in one person who is involved in a close relationship with another person who already has a delusional disorder. The primary individual is dominant in the relationship and gradually imposes his or her delusional system on the more passive and initially healthy second person" (Ellis, 2000, page 218). In DSM-IV-TR, *folie à deux* is called shared psychotic disorder.

Cognitive Dissonance

One of the most influential and powerful ideas in social psychology, cognitive dissonance theory posits that individuals experience a strong motivation to resolve inconsistencies in their thoughts, feelings, behavior, and circumstances. This concept was identified and investigated by Leon Festinger (1957, 1959). For example, a person forced to complete a dull, boring task with little reward will find inner justification for his or her actions. The anxiety or dissonance that an individual experiences in a coerced situation will often lead to the creation of reasons or justifications for remaining in the situation. Individuals holding opposite and contradictory views will often find it necessary to modify one belief or another, in order to resolve the logical inconsistency. Cognitive dissonance can lead to defense mechanisms such as denial and reversal.

Cognitive dissonance has generally been studied in adults, but recent research by Louisa C. Egan, Ph.D., and her colleagues has demonstrated the phenomenon of cognitive dissonance in young children and also capuchin monkeys. These authors commented that their research "raises the possibility that the drive to reduce dissonance is an aspect of human psychology that emerges without the need for much experience. Indeed, behavioral similarities between young human subjects and closely-related primates are a signature of cognitive systems that are typically thought to be constrained across development, maybe even emerging innately" (Egan et al., 2007).

The experience of cognitive dissonance helps to explain the phenomenon of parental alienation. The child presumably experiences a strong emotional connection to each of his or her parents, but finds the emotional connection to the alienating parent threatened by that parent's strong rejection of the other. Resolution of the inconsistency is achieved by the child's likewise rejecting the other parent. The phenomenon is accompanied by defensive techniques such as denial (as in refusing to acknowledge the positive attributes of the rejected parent), confirmatory bias (in generating manufactured reasons for the rejection), and reversal (actively seeking to accommodate the rejecting parent's wishes despite the child's initial, true feelings). The role of cognitive dissonance in the development of parental alienation was specifically studied by Uwe Jopt and Katharina Behrend and discussed in their papers, "Das Parental Alienation Syndrome (PAS)–Ein Zwei-Phasen-Modell" ("The parental alienation syndrome: A two-stage model") (German) (Jopt and Behrend, 2000a, 2000b).

False Memory Research

The extensive research of Stephen J. Ceci and his colleagues regarding childhood suggestibility and false memory formation shows that children are particularly susceptible to being influenced or led by others, even to create beliefs of events that have not actually occurred (Ceci and Bruck, 1993, 1995, 2006). As Richard Warshak pointed out, "Studies on memory, suggestibility, stereotype induction, social influence, and coercive influence demonstrate that children are susceptible to accepting, and repeating as if true, suggestions implanted by adult interviewers that innocent adults did harmful or illegal things" (Warshak, 2006). Children are much more susceptible to hypnotic influence than the average adult (Olness and Kohen, 1996). Thus, children are especially vulnerable to adopting the beliefs and feelings of a strong-willed adult, particularly if the adult is someone with whom they have a close emotional connection, such as a parent.

Parent Loss

In cases of severe parental alienation, the child loses her relationship with a loving parent for many years, perhaps a lifetime. There is abundant clinical experience and systematic research indicating that loss of a parent—whether by death, divorce, abandonment, chronic illness, or imprisonment—may have serious consequences for children. However, we believe that the loss of a parent through parental alienation may be more damaging than loss of a parent through death or abandonment. In the case of parental alienation, the child may become extremely confused and distraught because of persistent ambivalence toward the alienated parent. Subsequently, the child may feel extremely guilty because she contributed to the alienation by adopting false beliefs or making false allegations.

Years before he described PAS, Richard Gardner (1979) wrote a book chapter, "Death of a Parent," from a psychoanalytic point of view. Gardner explained the healthy mourning process in children (including grieving, anger, forming substitute relationships, and some forms of identification with the deceased parent) and pathological reactions to parental death (denial, guilt, suppression, repression, regression, depression, and pathological identification). Beardslee and Hoke (1997) studied the reaction of children to a parent's chronic illness, whether it be a mental disorder, such as a mood disorder, or a physical condition, such as cancer. They said, "A parental medical illness, like a psychiatric illness, affects children and families on multiple levels and places some children at increased risk for developing adjustment problems." They also emphasized the importance of resiliency in children and various prevention strategies. In cases of severe parental alienation, parentectomy occurs. The short-term and long-term consequences of parental alienation are discussed in Section 16 of this chapter.

Children's Rights

There have been many formal and informal declarations of children's rights, including statements by international and global organizations. In 1924, the League of Nations General Assembly endorsed a statement, the Declaration of the Rights of the Child, which consisted of five principles. In 1959, the United Nations General Assembly adopted a more elaborate statement with the same name, the Declaration of the Rights of the Child, which consisted of ten principles. Principle 6 stated: "The child, for the full and harmonious development of his personality, needs love and understanding. He shall, wherever possible, grow up in the care and under the responsibility of his parents, and, in any case, in an atmosphere of affection and of moral and material security; a child of tender years shall not, save in exceptional circumstances, be separated from his mother."

Thirty years later, in 1989, the United Nations established the Convention on the Rights of the Child (CRC), which consists of 54 sections or articles. The CRC has been signed and ratified by every country in the world except the United States. Several of the articles of the CRC relate to the problem of parental alienation. For example, Article 3 states: "In all actions concerning children, whether undertaken by public or private social welfare institutions, courts of law, administrative authorities or legislative bodies, the best interests of the child shall be a primary consideration" (United Nations Children's Fund, 2009, page 75). More directly, Article 18 states: "States Parties shall use their best efforts to ensure recognition of the principle that both parents have common responsibilities for the upbringing and development of the child. Parents or, as the case may be, legal guardians have the primary responsibility for the upbringing and development of the child. The best interests of the child will be their basic concern" (United Nations Children's Fund, 2009, page 77).

The Council of Europe, which was established in 1949, now includes 47 countries. In the following year, the European Convention on Human Rights (ECHR) was signed, and several protocols were subsequently added. In 1959, the European Court of Human Rights (ECtHR) was established to enforce the terms of the ECHR. The ECtHR, which meets in Strasbourg, France, typically hears cases in which a private citizen is suing his or her government because of an alleged deprivation of human rights. Article 8 of the ECHR states: "Everyone has the right to respect for his private and family life, his home and his correspondence." The ECtHR has handled cases involving child custody, visitation, and parental alienation when a parent alleged that his rights to have access his children were violated. See Appendix C, page 172, of this book for summaries of several instances in which the ECtHR considered cases involving parental alienation.

Emotional Abuse of Children

Although DSM-IV-TR provides diagnostic criteria for physical abuse of a child, sexual abuse of a child, and neglect of a child, there is thus far no diagnosis for the emotional component of abuse. However, ICD-10 does include "child emotional/psychological abuse" (T74.3). Emotional abuse has been studied, and the following categories of emotional abuse were proposed by Garbarino et al. (1986) and amended by Pearl (1994): rejecting the child; isolating the child from normal social experiences; terrorizing the child verbally and with threats of assault; ignoring the child; corrupting the child by encouraging antisocial behavior; berating the child; and overpressuring the child.

We agree with Johnston, who stated that parental alienation constitutes child abuse. She said, "With respect to the parents' need for mandated treatment, we argue that alienating behavior by parents is a malignant form of emotional abuse of children that needs to be corrected, whether a parent agrees or not. A growing body of literature on the adverse effects of parents' psychological control, also called 'intrusive parenting,' supports this contention" (Johnston, 2005).

Several other authors have stated that parental alienation should be considered psychological or emotional abuse of the child, including mental health professionals from Canada (Gagné and Drapeau, 2005), Germany (Boch-Galhau and Kodjoe, 2006b, and Deegener and Körner, 2005), Italy (Malagoli Togliatti and Franci, 2005, and Gulotta et al., 2008), Spain (Tejedor Huerta, 2007a), South Africa (Szabo, 2002), the United Kingdom (Lowenstein, 2007), and the United States

(Gardner, 1985, Warshak, 2001, Cartwright, 2006, and Baker, 2007). Hamarman and Bernet devised a way to stratify emotional abuse of children into mild, moderate, and severe levels. Given their definitions, many instances of parental alienation would meet the criteria for severe emotional abuse, which is "characterized by actions that inflict emotional harm and are performed with malicious intent" (Hamarman and Bernet, 2000).

Domestic Violence Research

Research on domestic violence indicates that some children become victims of parental coercive control and domination. In these families, a parent harasses and controls the former partner by manipulating the children to turn against the victim parent. Jaffe and his colleagues wrote, "Abusive ex-partners are likely to attempt to alienate the children from the other parent's affection (by asserting blame for the dissolution of the family and telling negative stories), sabotage family plans (by continuing criticism with competitive bribes), and undermine parental authority (by explicitly instructing the children not to listen or obey)" (Jaffe et al., 2008). The population of violent men who alienate their children from their mothers has also been studied by Berns et al. (1999), by Beeble et al. (2007) and by Drozd and Olesen (2004), who labeled alienating behavior by spousal abusers as "sabotage."

Children's Competency to Testify and Give Informed Consent

Competency refers to the child's ability to testify in court in a reliable, meaningful manner. Weissman (1991) summarized the four criteria that are generally required to establish competency: "the capacity to perceive facts accurately (e.g., mental capacity at the time of instant occurrence to observe or receive accurate impressions of the occurrence); the capacity to recollect and recall (e.g., memory sufficient to retain an independent recollection of the observation); the capacity to understand the oath (e.g., capacity to differentiate truth from falsehood, to comprehend the duty to tell the truth, and to understand the consequences of not fulfilling the duty); and the capacity to communicate based on personal knowledge of the facts (e.g., capacity to communicate the memory of such observation, and to understand simple questions about the occurrence)."

A child's competency may become an issue because it is common for children and adolescents to testify in trials related to their parents' custody and visitation disputes. Judges typically take into consideration the opinions and expressed preferences of older childen and adolescents. In some states, judges are required to allow the testimony of children older than a specified age, but the judges are not required to order what the youngster requests. In cases of alleged parental alienation, the attorney for the targeted parent may argue that the child is not competent to testify because he has been indoctrinated and is not expressing his true opinion. For example, his "capacity to recollect and recall" past events may be impaired because post-event suggestive and leading questions caused the child to adopt false memories.

A similar argument could be made regarding the child's ability to give informed consent. Although the criteria for informed consent may vary depending on the circumstances, the general rule is that informed consent must be: knowing (the person has sufficient information regarding the proposed course of action and the possible alternatives); intelligent (the person has rationally weighed the advantages and disadvantages of the various possibilities); and voluntary (the person has not been coerced to make a particular decision). In cases of alleged parental alienation, it could be argued that the child is not competent to express an opinion or make a decision regarding where she will live. That is, the indoctrination associated with the parental alienation constituted a form of coercion that prevented the child from rationally considering the pros and cons of living with one parent or the other.

This argument has been successful in cases in Europe. In the case of *C. v. Finland,* which was argued before the European Court of Human Rights in 2006, the parents divorced and subsequently the mother died. Although the father had custody of the children, they refused to see him. This case ultimately reached the European Court of Human Rights, which concluded that the children had been indoctrinated or manipulated to dislike the father. The legal issue was that the manipulated child's stated preference should not be accepted as his or her real desire, that is, the manipulated child is not competent to give informed consent. See Appendix C, page 172, of this book for more information about this case.

Family Systems Theory

Another strand of support for the existence of parental alienation comes from family systems theory. Family systems theorists have long identified parent-child alignment against the other parent as a significant problem in the structure and dynamics of the family. The concept of triangulation has been employed to great effect to explain the origin and maintenance of dysfunctional family relationships. Triangulation involves two members of a family drawing in or excluding a third family member. (The notion of "triangulation" as a dysfunctional family relationship is unrelated to the use of "methodological triangulation" as a research tool.) A common form of triangulation is cross-generational coalition, a phenomenon that many family therapists, including pioneers (e.g., Bowen, 1966, 1978; Kerr and Bowen, 1988; Minuchin, 1974) have linked to the development of maladjustment and children. According to Minuchin, cross-generational coalitions develop when one or both parents try to enlist the support of the child against the other parent. Confiding in the child, treating the child as a partner, and involving the child in adult disputes are all behaviors that typify cross-generational alliances. Parental alienation can easily be conceptualized as an extreme form of such a pathological coalition.

Psycholinguistic Analysis

In general, psycholinguistics refers to the study of psychological states and mental activity associated with the use of language. Psycholinguists study the relationship between language and thought. A group of Italian psychologists (Gulotta et al., 2008) have undertaken the psycholinguistic analysis of family members affected by parental alienation. In their recent book, *La Sindrome di Alienazione Parentale (PAS): Lavaggio del Cervello e Programmazione dei Figli in Danno Dell'altro Genitore (The Parental Alienation Syndrome [PAS]: Brainwashing and Programming of Children to the Detriment of the Other Parent)*, they described their method for identifying alienating behavior by carefully analyzing the dialogue among the family members. Their book contains many examples of the subtle and not-so-subtle messages that an alienating parent might communicate to a child. See an example in the case vignette on page 90.

Psycholinguistic Analysis Reveals Parental Alienation
Professor Guglielmo Gulotta, Turin, Italy

Prof. Gulotta has studied transcripts of children's statements as a way to investigate the phenomenon of parental alienation. He provided an example from an Italian case in which a father had been charged with abusing his daughter. In this case, a psychological consultant hired by the Court was skeptical regarding the allegations. In the following excerpt of the psychologist's interview, it is apparent that the girl was indoctrinated by her mother to dislike the father (Gulotta et al., 2008, page 11).

Psychologist: "Is your father always so bad?"
Little girl: "No, he isn't. Sometimes he calls me 'Sweetheart!'"
Psychologist: "Do you know why?"
Little girl: "Because then he can go home and say, 'I tricked her! Now she believes I love her, so the judge will give me custody and her mother will cry!'"
Psychologist: "But, do you love your father?"
Little girl: "Yes, I do. But do you know why I love him? The devil makes me love my father. So, I'll want to stay with him and my mother will be alone crying!"
Psychologist: "How do you know that?"
Little girl: "My Mom told me! I remember that my Mom and I made tape recordings in order to leave him. Actually, he was already moved, but in order to not have him back!"

Professor Gulotta, one of the contributors to this book, also cited a very short example of a destructive communication style, which was taken from court testimony. During a trial, the attorney questioned a mother as to whether she had influenced her son against the father. The mother replied, "Influence my son against his father?! But, we never even talk about him! It's as though he doesn't exist anymore!" The mother clearly explained—in her own way—that failure to talk about the father was a way to communicate negative opinions about him.

In-group, Out-group Phenomena

The importance of in-group and out-group phenomena has been studied by Cynthia L. Pickett, Marilynn B. Brewer (Pickett and

Brewer, 2005), and other social psychologists. The theory is that individuals require connectedness to others in order to maintain a positive sense of self. As a result, people are very inclined to adopt the beliefs and practices of a given social group that admits them. In some social situations, the sense of being included by members of an in-group is heightened by actively and energetically excluding members of an out-group. It is easy to see how a similar mechanism occurs when a child, who is motivated to be accepted by one parent, actively rejects the other parent.

Therapist Alienation

In psychotherapy, children and adolescents may resist talking to the therapist and participating in the treatment process for a number of different reasons. Disruption of the patient-therapist alliance is typically related to forces *within* the therapy dyad, e.g., the patient is defensive because he feels the therapist will dislike him or criticize him if he reveals his personal thoughts and feelings. However, Benjamin Garber has focused on the phenomenon of "therapist alienation," which occurs when family members *outside* the therapy dyad rupture the patient-therapist alliance. Garber considered therapist alienation to be a cousin of parental alienation. Garber explained that therapist alienation is sometimes obvious from the child's unambiguous statements, such as "Mommy told me not to talk to you" (Garber, 2004a). The phenomenon of therapist alienation (which the mental health professional directly observes) supports the reality of parental alienation (which the mental health professional may only hear about through collateral sources).

11. Systematic research indicates that the criteria used to diagnose PAS are reliable.

As explained previously, social researchers may use methodological triangulation—using a variety of research methods to address a particular question—in their studies, which enables them to overcome the weaknesses of using a single method of research. We previously summarized several types of qualitative research that were used to reach the conclusion that PAS is a valid concept. In this section we summarize two quantitative studies, which increase confidence that PAS can be reliably measured. This is an example of methodological triangulation. Regarding this approach, Webb et al. (1966) states "Once a proposition has been confirmed by two or more independent processes, the uncertainty of its interpretation is greatly reduced. The most pervasive evidence comes through a triangulation of measurement."

Reliability refers to the consistency of a test, survey instrument, observation, or other measuring device. For example, test-retest reliability refers to the test's consistency in measuring between different administrations. Inter-rater reliability refers to the degree of agreement between evaluators when evaluating the same phenomenon. There have been two test-retest and inter-rater reliability studies on PAS conducted and published, one in a peer-reviewed journal and one in the form of a dissertation. In these studies, the researchers measured the agreement of evaluators, using Gardner's definition of PAS, when presented with vignettes. High measures of agreement suggest reliability and low measures suggest the opposite. These two reliability studies, summarized here, represent quantitative research on PAS.

Carlos Rueda, Ph.D., and Inter-Rater Reliability

Carlos Rueda, Ph.D., conducted the first inter-rater reliability study on PAS. The concept of PAS examined was grounded in Gardner's conceptual framework, that is, the definition of PAS and eight defined symptoms. Rueda sent the survey instrument to doctoral level mental health professionals and asked each to examine five vignettes that related to PAS. The evaluation instrument was designed and created by "a panel of experts who were consulted on the study's language, instrumentation, methodology, and case selection." The vignettes used for the study were based on real-life scenarios.

Evaluators upon reading each vignette were asked to determine, "Did the scenario presented meet the criteria for PAS?" with the choice of answers being "No," "Not sure," and "Yes." Next, respondents were asked "Which type of PAS?" with the choice of answers being "Mild," "Moderate," or "Severe." In addition, each respondent was asked to assess a total of 23 questions based on Gardner's eight symptoms of PAS, including 10 questions regarding the parent behaviors and 13 questions regarding the child behaviors. In Rueda's study, 14 evaluators responded and participated in the test (the first sending of the vignettes) and 10 of the 14 completed the re-test (the same five vignettes sent 60 days later to the same respondents) (Rueda, 2003, 2004).

Rueda measured the degree of inter-rater reliability in two ways. First, he assessed whether evaluators were able to agree that PAS was or was not present and on the level of PAS, mild, moderate or severe. In this kind of study, researchers are able to measure the degree of agreement, from no agreement between evaluations to total agreement between evaluations. Kendall's Coefficient of Concordance (also called Kendall's W) was used to determine the degree of agreement among the evaluators. A zero obtained value indicates no agreement and a one obtained value indicates total agreement. A result of .60 is the minimum value suggesting agreement, although some researchers prefer .70 as a minimum acceptable value. The Kendall's W values obtained in the Rueda study are indicated in Table 1. There was a high rate of agreement among the evaluators, both for the test and the retest.

TABLE 1. KENDALL'S W VALUES FOR RUEDA'S
INTER-RATER RELIABILITY STUDY

	Vignette 1	*Vignette 2*	*Vignette 3*	*Vignette 4*	*Vignette 5*
Test	1.00	.889	.923	.909	.923
Retest	1.00	1.00	.889	1.00	1.00

Second, Rueda assessed whether evaluators were able to agree on the presence or absence of the eight symptoms of PAS. That is, whether they agreed regarding the 23 questions based on the eight symptoms of PAS, including 10 questions regarding the parent behaviors and 13 questions regarding the child behaviors. SPSS, a statistical software program, was used to obtain the intraclass correlation coefficient. Again, a zero obtained value indicates no agreement and a one obtained value indicates agreement, with .70 being the minimum values suggesting agreement. Table 2 presents the obtained intraclass correlation coefficient (alpha values) for each of the five vignettes. Rueda found a high rate of agreement regarding the diagnostic criteria for PAS. The results indicated reliability for Rueda's PAS test instrument in measuring or testing for PAS, based on Gardner's definition of PAS and eight defined symptoms.

TABLE 2. INTRACLASS CORRELATION COEFFICIENT
(ALPHA VALUES) FOR RUEDA'S INTER-RATER RELIABILIATY STUDY

	Vignette 1	*Vignette 2*	*Vignette 3*	*Vignette 4*	*Vignette 5*
Test	.9171	.9061	.8237	.7963	.6189
Retest	.9376	.8012	.8565	.8131	.8486

Stephen Morrison, Ph.D., and Inter-Rater Reliability

Stephen Morrison, Ph.D., conducted a second test-retest and inter-rater reliability study, an exact replication of Rueda (2003), using the same vignettes and PAS test instrument. This replication was designed in this way to make it possible to compare the results of the two studies. In the Morrison study, the survey instrument and vignettes were sent to child custody and mental health practitioners in the U.S., but not in Florida, the primary source of respondents for the Rueda study. (This was to minimize the potential for obtaining duplicate respondents.) In this study, 31 evaluators participated in the test (the first sending of the vignettes) and 20 of the 31 in the retest (the same vignettes sent 60 days later) (Morrison, 2006).

Morrison also measured the degree of inter-rater reliability in two ways. First, he assessed whether evaluators were able to agree that PAS was or was not present and on the level of PAS, mild, moderate or severe. The Kendall's W values obtained in the Morrison study are indicated in Table 3. The values obtained reflect agreement except on Vignette 2 and weak agreement on Vignette 4. There are several possible reasons for these findings. However, it is believed that this is because in Vignette 2 there were no symptoms of PAS and in Vignette 4 the symptoms were weak. This indicates the recognition difficulty evaluators have when PAS occurs in mild form. Of course, the assessment of the vignettes was conducted in a laboratory, which has limitations when compared to real life.

TABLE 3. KENDALL'S W VALUES FOR
MORRISON'S INTER-RATER RELIABILITY STUDY

	Vignette 1	*Vignette 2*	*Vignette 3*	*Vignette 4*	*Vignette 5*
Test	1.00	.346	.737	.684	.800
Retest	1.00	.296	.778	.778	.850

Second, Morrison also assessed whether evaluators were able to agree on the presence or absence of the eight symptoms of PAS. The results of this inter-rater reliability study are presented in Table 4. These obtained intraclass correlation coefficient values in Morrison's second inter-rater reliability study all approach one and indicate significant agreement among evaluators, especially in the vignettes where the symptoms are pronounced and/or visible. The results indicate the PAS test instrument is reliable when testing for PAS.

TABLE 4. INTRACLASS CORRELATION COEFFICIENT (ALPHA VALUES) FOR MORRISON'S INTER-RATER RELIABILITY STUDY

	Vignette 1	*Vignette 2*	*Vignette 3*	*Vignette 4*	*Vignette 5*
Test	.8117	.7787	.9471	.8910	.9251
Retest	.8515	.7992	.9493	.9033	.9169

Zirogiannis (2001), states "When a standardized test measures the occurrence of a disease or syndrome, the test is reliable if different evaluators giving the same test derive the same or similar conclusions." The collected high intraclass correlation coefficient values in both Rueda (2003, 2004) and Morrison (2006) indicate agreement and consensus among evaluators working independently. Both studies indicate the PAS test instrument is reliable for determining the presence and degree of PAS and is reliable when used to identify PAS based on Gardner's eight defined symptoms of PAS.

Test-Retest Reliability

In addition to assessing the inter-rater reliability of the instrument for identifying PAS, Rueda and Morrison also measured the test-retest reliability of the instrument. Test-retest reliability refers to the test's consistency in measuring between different administrations by the same evaluators. A test is deemed reliable if evaluators produce the same results when measuring the same subjects at different times. Of importance is the amount of time between tests. If the time period is too short, the evaluators' answers may be based on their memories of the first administration of the test. If the time period is too long, the evaluators may mature and their answers may be based on different and or newly acquired knowledge. In these two studies, a time period of 60 days elapsed between evaluations. The answers by each of the evaluators during the "test" were compared to their answers during the "retest."

In reporting the degree of test-retest reliability, Rueda said, "The second round concerning the retest began 60 days after the initial survey was sent and there was not much variation from the original observations. From the total number of questions answered by all respondents in all five cases, only 2.1 percent of the answers showed a slight variation in the second round" (Rueda, 2004). Morrison, one of the contributors to this book, reviewed his data and arrived at a similar conclusion. He said there were 2,666 questions that were answered during both the first and second administration of the questionnaires to the evaluators. Morrison said, "Of these 2,666 answered questions, 10.8 percent changed from the first to the second administration." The Rueda and Morrison studies indicate a high degree of test-retest reliability for the PAS test instrument.

12. It is possible to estimate the prevalence of parental alienation at 1% of children and adolescents in the U.S.

The prevalence of parental alienation has been studied. In general, parental alienation is more likely to occur in highly conflicted, custody-disputing families than in community samples of divorcing families. Even in highly conflicted divorces, only the minority of children experience parental alienation. The following studies indicate that approximately 25 percent of children involved in custody disputes manifest parental alienation. The exact number depends on: the researcher's definition of parental alienation; whether one considers all levels of parental alienation or only a severe degree of parental alienation; and whether the researchers distinguished alienation (unjustified rejection of the parent) and estrangement (justified rejected of the parent).

Janet Johnston, Ph.D.

Janet Johnston—in California—found that 7 percent of the children in one study and 27 percent of the children in a second study had "strong alignment" with one parent and rejection of the other parent (Johnston, 1993). Subsequently, Johnston reported that 15 percent of children in a community sample of divorcing families and 21 percent in contested custody cases experienced either "some" or "much" alignment with one parent or the other (defined as the "child's behavioral and verbal preference for one parent with varying degrees of overt or covert negativity toward other parent" (Johnston, 2003, 2005). In these statistics, Johnston did not distinguish whether the child's negativity toward the other parent was justified (because of domestic violence, for example) or unjustified. (We calculated these percentages using the raw data available in Johnston [2003] and found that 18 percent of the children in the community sample and 27 percent in the contested custody cases experienced some degree of alignment.)

Leona Kopetski, M.S.S.W.

Leona Kopetski–in Colorado–found that 20 percent of families involved in custody disputes manifested parental alienation syndrome (Kopetski, 1998a).

Larry Nicholas, Ph.D.

Larry Nicholas–in California–reported on a survey of 21 custody evaluators (Nicholas, 1997). According to Nicholas, the majority of respondents to his survey reported that in about one-third of their custody evaluation cases, one parent was engaging in identifiable alienating behavior.

Amy Baker, Ph.D.

Amy Baker–in New York–surveyed 106 mental health professionals who conducted custody evaluations. The respondents reported that PAS occurred in between 0 percent and 55 percent of their cases, with an average of 11.2 percent (SD = 13). Baker found that the evaluators who identified PAS more frequently were more familiar with the concept of PAS, were more likely to assess for PAS, were more likely to believe that one parent can turn a child against the other parent, and were more confident in their evaluations (Baker, 2007a).

James N. Bow, Ph.D., and Colleagues

James N. Bow, Jonathan W. Gould, and James R. Flens surveyed 448 mental health and legal professionals who were experienced with parental alienation. They said, "When respondents were asked [in] what percentage of child custody cases was parental alienation an issue, the mean reported was 26 percent (SD = 22), with a median of 20" (Bow et al., 2009).

The prevalence of parental alienation in the U.S. can be roughly estimated as follows. (1) In a recent report, the U.S. Census Bureau estimated that about 20 percent of children under age 18 live with separated or divorced parents (United States Census Bureau, 2009); (2) In approximately 20 percent of separations and divorces, there is serious disagreement involving the children, which sometimes leads to formal custody or visitation disputes (Hetherington and Kelly, 2002, page 138); and (3) As explained earlier in this section, when there is serious disagreement between parents regarding custody and visitation, approximately 25 percent of the children develop parental alienation. Multiplying these percentages yields a prevalence of 1 percent, or about 740,000 children and adolescents in the U.S. For comparison purposes, this prevalence is about the same as the prevalence of autism spectrum disorders among children and adolescents in the U.S.

We realize this is a very rough estimate, but it is probably the correct order of magnitude. When parental alienation is recognized as an official diagnosis and formal criteria are established, it will be possible to determine its prevalence more accurately. This estimate may be lower than the actual number of children and adolescents who experience parental alienation. In calculating this estimate, it was assumed that parental alienation only occurs in divorced families, while it may also occur in intact families. Also, many instances of parental alienation after divorce never come to the attention of the legal system because many targeted parents lose contact with their children and never fight about it in court because they do not have the resources or do not want to make the situation worse.

13. Parental alienation and PAS have been discussed by professional organizations.

American Academy of Child and Adolescent Psychiatry

In 1997, the American Academy of Child and Adolescent Psychiatry (AACAP) published "Practice Parameters for Child Custody Evaluations." This document, an "AACAP Official Action," referred explicitly to "Parental Alienation" and said, "There are times during a custody dispute when a child can become extremely hostile toward one of the parents. The child finds nothing positive in his or her relationship with the parent and prefers no contact. The evaluator must assess this apparent alienation and form a hypothesis of its origins and meaning. Sometimes, negative feelings toward one parent are catalyzed and fostered by the other parent; sometimes, they are an outgrowth of serious problems in the relationship with the rejected parent" (American Academy of Child and Adolescent Psychiatry, 1997b).

Licensed Clinical Social Workers

In 2005, Virginia H. Luftman, M.S.W., and her colleagues published "Practice Guidelines in Child Custody Evaluations for Licensed Clinical Social Workers." These guidelines discuss a number of topics including ethical considerations, the parent-child relationship, parenting style, gender issues, parental conflict, and parental alienation. After explaining Gardner's definition of PAS, they said, "Although there is implicit professional consensus that one parent has the capacity to influence children negatively against the other parent, there are those who do not classify this rejection as a 'syndrome.' . . . Regardless, it is important for the evaluator to address each parent's acceptance of a child's need to be co-parented and their acknowledgment of the importance of the child's attachment to the other parent. Any attempts by one parent to disrupt the relationship of the child to the other parent should be duly noted and included in the report to the court" (Luftman et al., 2005).

American Psychological Association

The American Psychological Association has addressed the topic of parental alienation on a number of occasions. In 1994, the American Psychological Association published "Guidelines for Child Custody Evaluations in Divorce Proceedings." The text of the guidelines does not refer explicitly to parental alienation, but simply states that the psychological assessment should include "an evaluation of the interaction between each adult and child" (American Psychological Association, 1994). However, the authors of the guidelines provided a highly selective bibliography (39 references) of "Pertinent Literature," which includes *The Parental Alienation Syndrome* and two other books by Richard Gardner, both of which include discussions about PAS. In 2009, the American Psychological Association published a revision to their 1994 document, which was called "Guidelines for Child Custody Evaluations in Family Law Proceedings" (American Psychological Association, 2009). The 2009 APA document cites several general principles for forensic evaluators (such as, "The purpose of the evaluation is to assist in determining the psychological best interests of the child"), but does not address specific methodology and topics to consider in conducting the evaluation.

In 1996, the American Psychological Association Presidential Task Force on Violence and the Family published a report, in which the authors expressed the concern that testimony regarding parental alienation might be misused. The Presidential Task Force report said, "Family courts often do not consider the history of violence between the parents in making custody and visitation decisions. In this context, the nonviolent parent may be at a disadvantage, and behavior that would seem reasonable as a protection from abuse may be misinterpreted as a sign of instability. Psychological evaluators not trained in domestic violence may contribute to this process by ignoring or minimizing the violence and by giving inappropriate pathological labels to women's responses to chronic victimization. Terms such as 'parental alienation' may be used to blame the women for the children's reasonable fear or anger toward their violent father" (American Psychological Association, 1996, page 100).

In January 2008, the American Psychological Association released an updated statement, as follows: "The American Psychological Association has no official position on 'parental alienation syndrome.' This concept has been used in contested child custody cases and has become the subject of significant debate. While it may be that in some divorces, children become estranged from their noncustodial parent for a variety of reasons, there is no evidence within the psychological literature of a diagnosable parental alienation syndrome" (American Psychological Association, 2008).

The problem with these succinct statements by the American Psychological Association is that they are ambiguous and perhaps misleading precisely because of their brevity. They are ambiguous for the following reasons: (1) These statements apparently are referring specifically to *parental alienation syndrome* (that is, including the "alienating parent" and the eight symptoms described by Richard Gardner), not to the more general notion of *parental alienation.* There is much more evidence to support the reality of parental alienation than for PAS. (2) In the reference to being "diagnosable," the authors from the American Psychological Association do not distinguish between the diagnosis of a "mental disorder" and the diagnosis of a "relational problem." As explained earlier in this book, both of these entities are diagnoses in the DSM, although the criteria for being a relational problem are much more relaxed than those for a mental disorder. (3) It is hard to know what these authors meant when they flatly said, "There is *no evidence* within the psychological literature. . . ." As related in this book, there is extensive qualitative research and a modest amount of quantitative research regarding both parental alienation and PAS in peer-reviewed journals and in book chapters and books. We understand how it might be argued that there is not enough quantitative research for PAS to be considered a mental disorder in DSM (a rather high threshold). However, there is abundant qualitative and quantitative research for parental alienation to be considered a relational problem (a rather low threshold). The 1996 and 2008 statements by the American Psychological Association do not address any of these nuances, and are not particularly helpful in this discussion of whether parental alienation should be included in DSM-5.

14. Parental alienation and PAS have been discussed extensively by legal professionals, including attorneys, trial courts, appellate courts, and supreme courts.

There is a common misunderstanding that there is a disclaimer somewhere in DSM-IV-TR that states that the DSM should not be used in legal settings. Although there is no such disclaimer, the authors of DSM-IV-TR did say, "There are significant risks that diagnostic information will be misused or misunderstood. These dangers arise because of the imperfect fit between the questions of ultimate concern to the law and the information contained in a clinical diagnosis" (American Psychiatric Association, 2000, pages xxxii-xxxiii). For example, they pointed out, "A diagnosis does not carry any necessary implications regarding the causes of the individual's mental disorder," and, "The fact that an individual's presentation meets the criteria for a DSM-IV diagnosis does not carry any necessary implication regarding the individual's degree of control over the behavior that may be associated with the disorder" (American Psychiatric Association, 2000, page xxxiii). The authors of DSM-IV-TR concluded their discussion of this topic on a positive note: "When used appropriately, diagnoses and diagnostic information can assist decision makers in their determinations" (American Psychiatric Association, 2000, page xxxiii). We—the authors of this book—believe that inclusion of parental alienation in DSM-5 will greatly assist attorneys and judges in making rational decisions regarding children of divorced parents.

The world of jurisprudence faces many different burdens and abilities of proof. In some types of cases, the judge and jury can study the physical evidence and listen to individuals who witnessed the event. Other parts of law do not benefit from occurrences so easily defined. The evidence is harder to interpret and the only witnesses are all interested parties. Sometimes it is argued that the actual injury that is claimed does not even exist in the natural world. Such a condition is parental alienation. What is parental alienation? What evidences it? What does it mean in practice? What can we do about it? These are the questions which must be addressed by the legal profession, who in turn look to the writings of mental health professionals—including the DSM—to provide guidance.

Judges and attorneys are charged with the duty to be able to fully understand, to nearly expert level, any variety of matters that comes before them. One day, they may need to decide whether a tire's sidewall construction was within industry standards and, if not, whether such deviation caused a crash. The next day the court may need to understand whether a child is resisting a parent because of overt mistreatment by one parent or subtle mistreatment by the other parent or the child's attempting to please one parent over the other. These are complex problems that are hard to define and understand without specific guidance from the psychological community. Clearly there are few, if any, people who can attain and retain the vast encyclopedia of knowledge required to address all tasks at law. It is perhaps with these realities in mind that the courts welcome and rely upon expert witnesses to help explain the technical subject matter under consideration. Specific criteria are set forth by which a court must qualify an expert, especially when the theory being advanced is not yet widely accepted in the legal community. With regard to psychological issues, the courts frequently look to the DSM. For this reason, American courts are paralyzed by the DSM's silence regarding parental alienation.

The courts understand their inability, as scientific laypeople, to differentiate emerging science from quack science. Thus, rather than give each party full leeway to bring in any expert witness and theory they wish, the courts lay out a clear blueprint of what evidence may be considered. These guidelines primarily descend from two landmark cases:

1. *Frye v. United States* (293 F. 1013 [D.C. Cir. 1923]) concerned a defendant subjected to a systolic blood pressure deception test. A change in blood pressure was claimed to prove his guilt. On appeal, the *Frye* test emerged: Before a new scientific principle or discovery can be used as evidence, it "must be sufficiently established to have gained general acceptance in the particular field in which it belongs." The *Frye* Test is often referred to as the general acceptance test.

2. In *Daubert v. Merrell Dow* (509 U.S. 579 [1993]) the Supreme Court of the United States found a need to put greater focus on the reliability of the theory. The *Daubert* test incorporates many considerations, including (a) whether the theory or technique can be and has been tested, (b) whether it has been subjected to peer review and publication, (c) its known or potential error rate, (d) the existence and maintenance of standards controlling its operations, and (e) whether it has attracted widespread acceptance within a relevant scientific community.

In the U.S., most states have adopted some version of *Daubert* or *Frye*. Whether it is *Frye's* "general acceptance in the particular field" or *Daubert's* "peer review" and "widespread acceptance within a relevant scientific community," the courts have essentially said the answer to questions like parental alienation will come not from the legal field but the mental health field. Basically, Daubert is used more often to exclude the presentation of unqualified evidence or what is called "junk science," which sometimes leads to the exclusion of parental alienation and PAS as topics for legal consideration. The courts sit waiting patiently for DSM-5 to provide necessary scientific guidance. It is of critical importance to American jurisprudence that the American Psychiatric Association take a position regarding parental alienation through DSM-5. In light of the overwhelming evidence,

Parentectomy by Judicial Action
Randy Warren, J.D., San Rafael, California

In this case, the mother abruptly moved with her two children (15-year-old Judy and 10-year-old Jimmy) out of the family residence. The children refused to see their father. When the father brought a custody motion, Judy suddenly claimed that he had inappropriately touched her. Judy also told Jimmy about the alleged touching, who began telling his schoolmates that his father had raped his sister.

As time passed, there were many manifestations of parental alienation. At Jimmy's first supervised visit with his father, the mother warned the supervisor *in the presence of the child* that the father "is a bad man." During the supervised visit, Jimmy verbally assaulted his father, calling him "a bad man" and using terms uncommon for a young boy, such as, "You don't know how to love." When Jimmy met with the custody evaluator, he recalled everything in black and white: the father was evil and the mother was perfect. The mother and both children each selected the same anecdotes to tell the evaluator, and even used identical, unusual words within a given story. The children had been, until their parents separated, very close to their paternal grandparents. After the separation, Judy and Jimmy became blatantly hostile to these grandparents, telling them never to contact them again.

There was considerable additional information consistent with parental alienation and false allegations against the father. For example, a witness described sitting in on all-night coaching sessions between the mother and Judy in which stories against the father were crafted. Also, the father was tested by an expert polygrapher, who reported a "greater than 99 percent" probability that the father was truthful in stating he had no inappropriate contact with his daughter. Finally, Judy's diary surfaced. It contained neither abuse references nor any darkness. Three psychologists read the diary, each separately finding it highly unlikely that its writer was being molested. The abuse claims that Judy made to police, teachers, her mother, and the custody evaluator were contradictory.

Although the court ordered reunification therapy for Jimmy and his father, the boy would not cooperate. At that point, Jimmy could not believe his father and simultaneously believe Judy, to whom he was very close. He experienced cognitive dissonance. No attempt was made to reunite Judy and her father. The case ended suddenly when the judge, citing his personal history as a prosecutor, said the children had suffered enough. The judge did not simply deny the father's supervised visitation with his children, but cut off the father's contact with both Judy and Jimmy forever. This case illustrates how important it is for both mental health professionals and legal professionals to have a good understanding of parental alienation.

DSM-5 should recognize parental alienation as a diagnosis.

The topics of parental alienation and PAS are frequently introduced, discussed, and debated in American courts. However, the silence of DSM over the years has resulted in inconsistent rulings regarding parental alienation in many jurisdictions (Lorandos, 2006a). This is a serious problem because consistency is one of the foundations of the public's trust in the law. A society must have clear, consistent guiding principles. Many courts, clearly uncomfortable when faced with DSM's silence regarding parental alienation and PAS, have found ways to rule on cases while totally ignoring the most important question that is before them. When courts choose to address the issues of parental alienation and PAS, there is no consistency in their rulings. When there is no standard of scientific agreement, courts may base their decisions on personal prejudices and biases.

LEGAL CASES

Some courts have accepted the scientific basis for parental alienation and PAS.

For example, Judge Hurtubise in Quebec Superior Court addressed PAS head-on, finding, "There appears to be sufficient evidence to suggest that the issue of Parental Alienation Syndrome (PAS) . . . needs to be seriously taken into consideration." The court went on to discuss six characteristics of PAS and apply them to the facts of the case in a logical and orderly manner (*R.F. v. S.P.* [2000] Q.J. No 3412, No 500-12-250739-004).

In Ontario, Canada, the Gardner definition of PAS is "the definition generally accepted in the psychology community" (*Pettenuzzo-Deschene v. Deschene* [2007] O.J. No. 3062).

Also, a judge in Florida said, "I find that parental alienation syndrome has passed the *Frye* test in my courtroom" (*Kilgore v. Boyd,* Circuit Court of the 13th Judicial Circuit, Hillsborough County, Florida).

In Illinois, a trial court held a *Frye* hearing and ruled that PAS had gained general acceptance in the field of psychology. However, that court made its final ruling using the traditional standard of "best interests of the child," so it did not need to incorporate PAS in its ruling.

On appeal, that state's supreme court declined to rule specifically on admissibility of PAS (In re Marriage of De Bates [2004] 819 N.E.2d 714).

Some courts have rejected the scientific basis for parental alienation and PAS.

When this occurs, courts commonly cite that parental alienation and PAS are not included in DSM. In a New York case, for instance, the court noted that PAS is not a syndrome approved by the American Psychiatric Association and it is not a psychiatric diagnosis in DSM-IV (*J.F. v. L.F.* [1999] 694 NYS 2d 592).

A similar conclusion was reached by an Alabama appellate court that if it reached the question, it would reject PAS under a *Frye* test because PAS was not listed in DSM-IV (*C.J. L. v. M.W.B.* [2003] 868 So.2d 451).

Thus, the courts of three states–Florida, Illinois, and Alabama– applied the *Frye* test to similar sets of facts yet came up with different conclusions. The authors of this book believe that DSM-5 should address the issue of parental alienation to help alleviate the confusion in the legal marketplace.

Some courts have avoided altogether making a decision regarding the scientific basis for parental alienation and PAS.

For example, a court in Arkansas used typical language when not ruling on PAS one way or the other: "We do not address the acceptability of this theory as a diagnostic theory" (*Jennifer Linder [Johnson] v. Deron Johnson,* CA 06-033 [2006] Ark. App. Lexis 780).

Or, a court might make a distinction between parental alienation and PAS, and accept one concept but not the other. In Connecticut, for example, the appellate court found that the trial court made a factual finding of parental alienation rather than relying on PAS, an "alleged psychiatric disorder" not listed in DSM-IV. The appellate court therefore made no ruling on PAS (*Ruggiero v. Ruggiero* [2003] 819 A.2d 864).

The lack of a consistent foundation leads to legal fuzziness, and opposite or contradictory results may occur. In Connecticut, for example, a child may not suffer from PAS because the court found no credible evidence of PAS in any scientific studies or peer-reviewed scientific literature (*Snyder v. Cedar* [2006] Lexis 520). However, that same child may well suffer from PAS if he or she were in Ohio, where a court found evidence of severe PAS, and as a result awarded full legal custody to the target parent (*Doerman v. Doerman* [2002] Lexis 3183). We find courts using estrangement (a general term for contact refusal) and alienation (contact refusal without legitimate justification) as though they are interchangeable conditions. There is a proper and logical evidentiary process that many courts can utilize once PAS is shown to meet the *Daubert* and *Frye* requirements. But as noted, many judges are unwilling to venture to go where the DSM will not.

Ultimately, the most important and prophetic words come from Canada, where the judge ruled that "evidence about PAS was interesting, and I suspect we in the court system may be hearing more about it in the future, particularly in child custody proceedings" (*R. v. K.C.* [2002] O.J. No. 3162). Indeed, these cases are becoming more commonplace in the courtrooms of America and Canada, especially when alienation often rewards the alienating parent. See Appendix C of this book for a list of cases in the U.S., Canada, and other countries in which parental alienation or PAS has been an issue.

Courts will see this issue more and more in the future. As jurists deal with this emotionally charged and critically important topic, they will turn their eyes to the most reliable source, DSM-5, the one source ratified by both the *Frye* and *Daubert* tests. The legal profession needs DSM-5 to take a stand, to tell the courts that the mental health profession considers parental alienation to be a valid diagnosis. Once the diagnosis is established, the courts will also ask mental health professionals how to treat alienation and what to do with children caught in the trap of parental alienation. Although this book focuses on what the mental health community can do to help judges and attorneys deal with parental alienation, there will also need to be changes within the legal system. In a recent article, Hon. Donna J. Martinson, a judge on the Supreme Court of Yukon Territory, Canada, suggested that part of the problem is that inexperienced generalist judges have difficulty with high-conflict cases. Judge Martinson (2010) concluded, "Unless the litigation is properly managed by specialist judges, the justice system unintentionally causes harm to children."

LAW REVIEW ARTICLES

"Law reviews" are the primary forum for academic publishing in the legal field. Law reviews commonly influence the development of legislation and are also cited by courts as a source of authority when reaching decisions on individual cases. Law reviews are widely accessible and indexed in major computerized databases such as LEXIS-NEXIS and Westlaw. As of July 2005, parental alienation had been referenced in at least 112 law reviews (Hoult, 2006). As of September 2009, a search of the LEXIS-NEXIS database of United States law reviews on the keyword phrase "parental alienation" produced 230 hits. Adding Canadian and United Kingdom journals to the search added 21 more hits.

The substantial attention devoted by law journals to the topic of parental alienation demonstrates that this is a subject of considerable interest and controversy in the legal community. This literature is highly polarized in the expressed opinions, with some authors strongly criticizing and other authors strongly supporting the concepts of parental alienation and PAS. Of course, the literature regarding parental alienation primarily relates to family law and legal contexts associated with family and domestic litigation. However, parental alienation has been addressed in other legal contexts such as criminal responsibility.

For example, there have reportedly been several instances in which a child under the influence of PAS shot and killed the alienated parent. There has been debate as to whether PAS should be admissible as part of the child's mental-state defense. April J. Walker, a law professor, discussed the 2004 murder of Richard Lohstroh, M.D., by his 10-year-old son. Walker said, "Many believed that the Lohstroh boy was suffering from the effects of PAS at the time he shot and killed his father," and she concluded that the child was a candidate for the insanity defense. She commented, "PAS is widely accepted in family courts and there has been a wealth of research on the subject" (Walker, 2006). In this regard, an important research question is the extent to which parental alienation may overlap with and/or be differentiated from other conditions, such as a delusional disorder focused on persecutory beliefs held by a child about a parent. The diagnostic task of identifying when rejection of a parent by child is "without legitimate justification" resembles the task of identifying when a nonbizarre belief warrants the diagnosis of delusional disorder.

Because of the *Frye* and *Daubert* tests in the United States, it is not surprising that law reviews have focused on questions such as whether parental alienation is generally accepted in the professional community, whether it can be or has been scientifically tested, whether it has been the subject of peer-reviewed scientific publication, and whether its diagnosis has a known or potential error rate. There is an obvious overlap between that type of inquiry and the present proposal of parental alienation as a candidate for inclusion in DSM-5. Law reviews have also focused on scientific questions of causation, outcome, and prognosis, which may factor heavily in a court's decision-making. How accurately can the causes of parental alienation be determined? To what extent is parental alienation harmful? Can parental alienation be prevented or reversed? Are the best interests of an alienated child different from those of a nonalienated child? Research regarding these intriguing questions will be possible after the mental health community agrees on the definition of parental alienation and the criteria for its diagnosis.

15. Parental alienation and PAS have been discussed extensively by the general public.

The discussion of parental alienation and PAS has not been confined to professional conferences and academic debate. A parental alienation storyline has been featured in prime time television (*Law & Order SVU,* "Alien," 2007), a recent Brazilian documentary (*Fading Away,* 2009), celebrity books (for example, *A Promise to Ourselves,* by Alec Baldwin, 2008), and heartfelt personal memoirs (for example, *The Parentectomy,* by Kimber Adams, 2009). These works—both fact and fiction—reflect the public's recognition of an issue that affects thousands of children, parents, and extended family members every year.

The public's response to parental alienation has been to educate each other and to advocate for children and targeted parents who have lost the loving relationships that they previously enjoyed. Individuals affected by parental alienation, as well as legal and mental health professionals, rely on both traditional and emerging media to understand and address the factors that lead a child to align with one parent and reject a relationship with the other parent. These individuals have also

Tragic Outcome of False Allegations
Robert A. Evans, Ph.D., Palm Harbor, Florida

A young father had two stepchildren, whom he raised as his own, and two biological children. After his divorce, he became alienated from his stepchildren. When the father told his former spouse that he wanted custody of his biological children in a postdivorce action, he was accused of sexually molesting his stepchildren. The father ultimately went to trial to face criminal charges of child abuse. Although there were serious contradictions in the stories of the alleged victims, the government prosecuted the case. The father realized the trial was not going well for him and he anticipated a sentence of 300 years in prison. Sadly, the father hanged himself the day before the verdict was announced. Posthumously, he was found guilty of 13 counts of lewd and lascivious behavior with minor children. The alienating mother told the children he died in a car accident.

contributed their personal experiences and perspectives to television, film, radio, books, and articles. Through the Internet, the general public has participated in social networking websites and online support and advocacy groups to educate others and increase the visibility of an issue that they consider very important. It is obvious that the general public considers parental alienation a real and serious phenomenon that affects many families and causes considerable distress and heartbreak.

See Appendix D of this book for an extensive list of books, films, television and radio shows, Internet sites, and support groups that address parental alienation. The citations from various media in Appendix D were originally developed for the general public, not mental health or legal professionals.

16. Parental alienation is a serious mental condition. It has a predictable course that often continues into adulthood and can cause serious, long-term, psychological problems.

There are several areas and types of research that relate to the temporal course of this condition, parental alienation, which will be summarized here. First, classic research regarding attachment by pioneers such as John Bowlby, Harry Harlow, and Mary Ainsworth. Second, informal studies regarding the course and outcome of parental alienation by mental health professionals who have published anecdotal observations. Third, systematic qualitative and quantitative research.

We are concerned that some writers have (1) trivialized and minimized the condition and its serious, long-term detrimental effects on both the children and the parents; (2) characterized parental alienation as an expectable and minor consequence of divorce; (3) misrepresented and/or distorted the existing scientific data regarding parental alienation; and (4) even denied the existence of parental alienation, a position that is utterly untenable given the existing clinical reports and research studies. We believe that Judith Wallerstein and Sandra Blakeslee are misinformed when they say, "Although the parent under attack may feel like the problem will never end, I've never seen an alignment last through adolescence" (Wallerstein and Blakeslee, 2003, page 243). Of course, these authors may be describing accurately their own clinical experience, but it is not consistent with many articles and book chapters written by mental health professionals who have studied and treated children, adolescents, and "adult children" affected by parental alienation. The authors of this book believe that parental alienation is a serious condition that causes considerable morbidity and in some cases can even be life-threatening. How many mental disorders that are already in the DSM result in the total loss of a child's relationship with a parent for many years, perhaps a lifetime?

RESEARCH REGARDING CHILD DEVELOPMENT

The importance of attachment as a fundamental component of healthy parent-child relationships has been firmly established in the literature of child development. The seminal literature regarding attachment and child development will be summarized here, though the present discussion is intended only as a brief introduction.

In the 1950s John Bowlby (1988), a British psychiatrist, worked with children who had been separated from their mothers and endeavored to define the bond between parent and child created during infancy and early childhood. Bowlby found that children separated from their parents failed to thrive and he developed the theory of attachment, which suggests that a special relationship or bond is formed between the child and the caregiver. This emotional attachment creates the foundation or model of the child's relationships with other individuals and influences the child's personality development. Bowlby also concluded that children separated from the caregiver experience short-term and possibly long-term negative effects on their cognitive and emotional life.

Harry Harlow, an American psychologist, wanted to see if Bowlby's theory of attachment could be demonstrated empirically. Harlow (1958) observed baby rhesus monkeys that were taken from their birth mothers and raised in isolation. These monkeys failed to thrive and apparently were severely disturbed psychologically. Harlow also placed baby rhesus monkeys in cages with wire surrogate parents (that provided food) and soft terrycloth surrogate parents (that did not provide food). Although the baby monkeys approached the wire parent when they wanted food, they preferred the warmth and nurturing of the terrycloth parent. Harlow thought his research suggested the importance of the parent-child relationship for healthy development.

Mary Ainsworth (1978) conducted research that was based on Bowlby's theory of attachment. She developed a way for the theory to be empirically tested, that is, the Strange Situation Protocol, a method for assessing and documenting separation and reunion behavior of young children. She described three patterns of attachment behavior: secure attachment, anxious-avoidant insecure attachment, and anxious-ambivalent insecure attachment. There has been considerable interest in studying whether these early patterns are related to subsequent psychological or behavioral problems as the children grow.

We are not suggesting that parental alienation is exactly the same as the maternal loss that Bowlby described or the sensory isolation experienced by Harlow's monkeys. We are simply pointing out that a healthy attachment to caregivers is an extremely important feature of normal human development and that parental alienation can severely compromise a child's ability to form normal, healthy attachments. Among other things, parental alienation destroys the healthy relationship the child previously had with the targeted parent. Parental alienation also perverts the child's relationship with the preferred parent. As stated earlier in this book, parental alienation might be conceptualized as a "disorder of attachment," along with mental disorders such as reactive attachment disorder and separation anxiety disorder.

INFORMAL, ANECDOTAL OBSERVATIONS

There is considerable anecdotal evidence that parental alienation causes both short-term and long-term consequences, ranging from minor distress to major psychopathology. For example, Douglas Darnall (1998, page 6) said, "Various studies have shown that youngsters exposed to even mildly alienating behaviors may have trouble learning, concentrating, relaxing, or getting along with their peers. They have been known to develop physical symptoms, such as severe headaches, and serious behavior problems. Alienation will have lasting effects on your children, even into adulthood." Also, Ludwig Lowenstein (2007, pages 39–40) reported that children who experienced PAS may manifest the following symptoms: anger; loss or a lack of impulse control; loss of self-confidence and self-esteem; clinging and separation anxiety; fears and phobias; depression and suicidal ideation; sleep disorder; and other symptoms.

The most comprehensive book regarding PAS is *The International Handbook of Parental Alienation Syndrome* (Gardner et al., 2006). In the chapter called "Future Predictions on the Fate of PAS Children: What Hath Alienators Wrought?," Richard Gardner (2006b) suggested that PAS children are likely to manifest the following mental disorders either during childhood or as adults: conduct disorder; psychopathy; separation anxiety disorder; dissociative disorder; delusional disorder; narcissistic personality disorder; and gender identity problems. In the chapter called "Psychological Consequences of PAS Indoctrination for Adult Children of Divorce and the Effects of Alienation on Parents," Wilfrid von Boch-Galhau and Ursula Kodjoe (2006b) noted, "The child's loyalty conflict is exacerbated. Of paramount significance in the emergence of the child's symptoms are fear, dependence, and identification with the alienator. Related psychodynamics can be found, for example, in the Stockholm syndrome, after kidnappings, or in cults." In the same book, Glenn Cartwright (2006) said, "The awful outcome of PAS is the complete separation of a child or children from a parent. Even more dreadful is that it is deliberately caused, maliciously done, and entirely preventable. This terrible form of child abuse has long-lasting and devastating effects for all concerned; the child not only loses a parent but is cheated of remembering that parent fondly, the lost parent anguishes over the loss of a child and is chronically haunted by the child's seeming rejection and hatred, and even the alienator's short-term victory is diminished by potential future guilt and possible lifelong backlash from the child."

In general, clinicians and researchers have said that parental alienation harms the child through the following mechanisms: the preferred parent uses strategies that are emotionally abusive; the preferred parent encourages the child to be cruel and ungrateful; the preferred parent encourages black-and-white thinking; the experience of parental alienation undermines critical thinking skills and problem solving; by totally cutting off unwanted people, parental alienation constitutes a poor role model for interpersonal relationships; parental alienation creates a negative self-image as the child comes to hate half of who he is; the process of parental alienation encourages the child to cut off aspects of his own self that resemble the alienated parent; the child loses numerous secondary relationships, i.e., the family of the alienated parent; and the experience of parental alienation encourages dependency on the preferred parent and undermines the child's sense of self-sufficiency

As a result of these interpersonal and intrapsychic processes, the child victim of parental alienation may develop the following types of problems:

- Poor self-image and low self-esteem: as a result of rejecting an innocent targeted parent, a child may experience long-term guilt and other negative thoughts and feelings.
- Anxiety and depression: given that alienated children have been forced to choose one parent over another—and are thus in a no-win, double-bind situation—it is not surprising that clinicians have reported anxiety and depression in this group. Suicidal ideation may occur, and completed suicides have been reported.
- Trust issues: a child who cannot trust his or her own parents is likely to have difficulty trusting others, thus undermining future relationships.
- Dependency and self-sufficiency issues: a child who has been forced to conform to the expectations and pressures of an alienating parent is likely to become overly dependent on that parent.
- Fears of abandonment: a child who experiences the loss of a targeted parent, perhaps with the extended family of the targeted parent, may become insecure about future relationships.
- Intimacy issues: a child who is forced to reject a beloved parent

may well have difficulty forming and maintaining intimate relationships with future partners.

- Impairment of cognitive and thinking skills: since the child has
been forced to accept the preferred parent's distorted view of reality, the child may fail to develop independent thinking and critical reasoning skills. This is commonly associated with "black and
white thinking," i.e., the alienating parent is seen as "all good"
and the targeted parent is seen as "all bad."

- Pathological and dysfunctional personality trait and tendencies:
these include impaired insight and judgment, feelings of helpless-
ness and hopelessness, entitlement problems, inappropriate anger
and rage, problems with impulse control, oppositional and defiant behavior, critical and manipulative behavior, and sociopathic
behavior (such as cruel behavior, a lack of empathy, and a lack of
remorse). These undesirable personality traits arise because
obsessed alienators tend to be poor role models and they teach
their children dysfunctional and maladaptive ways of thinking,
feeling, and acting, particularly with respect to family and other
interpersonal relationships.

Not only does the child victim of parental alienation experience
serious psychological consequences, but the rejected, alienated parent
is also damaged. At the outset of parental alienation, the rejected parent is typically puzzled, then confused, and then extremely frustrated
as he or she tries to re-establish the nurturing relationship that the parent previously enjoyed with the child. The alienated parent is likely to
be criticized no matter what he or she does. If the rejected parent with-
draws to "give the child space," the parent is accused of being disin-
terested. If the rejected parent insists on having contact with the child,
the parent is accused of being insensitive and intrusive. The rejected
parent may become very angry and very depressed. The rejected parent may face the stressors of false allegations of abuse, the prospect of
conviction and incarceration, incompetent therapists, misguided
lawyers, and a painfully slow, counterproductive legal system.

A Young Woman Damaged by Her Father's Absence
Ursula Kodjoe, M.A., Emmendingen/Freiburg, Germany

Ms. Kodjoe, a psychologist and mediator, had a family meeting with a young woman, age 18, and her father. The daughter, who was trying to reverse the parental alienation she experienced most of her life, requested the meeting. The father and daughter wanted to talk.

The girl was 6 years old when her parents separated. She related that she only remembered her parents fighting. She said she was scared to lose her father and she lost him. She met him a few times after court hearings. The judge's orders were not followed. The girl's mother decided she only needed to see her father if she really wanted to.

By the time of the meeting, the daughter experienced no attachment, no connectedness, no inner relationship with her father. She felt no safety, no closeness. The daughter was overburdened by these feelings. For years, she did not dare express her longing for her father. At times, she did not know whether she wanted to see him or not. She kept wondering whether he wanted to see her and whether he remembered her.

In the meeting with Ms. Kodjoe, the daughter started crying and said her father never looked at the room she had as a child and he never even entered her home. The father sadly responded that he couldn't, he wasn't allowed, he was legally forbidden. The girl said, "If you loved me, you would have come anyway."

The daughter said she hated her father for accepting her mother's conditions. She hated her mother for burying her father alive. His name was never mentioned in the mother's home. The daughter thought she did not meet her father's expectations. She felt guilty, enraged, abandoned, anxious, and sad. The father thought he did not meet his daughter's expectations of closeness, protection, safety, and fatherhood. He felt guilty, enraged, powerless, and helpless.

The girl related to Ms. Kodjoe that on the day she turned 18, she ran away from her mother's home and dropped out of school. She wanted to go on with school somehow, but did not know how. The girl said that when she was 14, she started having sexual relationships with both boys and older men. Tearfully, she said she planned to live with a man twice her age, who was just like her father, unreliable and irresponsible.

The daughter realized that every important relationship failed because of her obsessive clinging. She was aware that she needed, requested, and demanded far too much attention. She could not do otherwise. This case clearly illustrates the serious, long-term consequences of parental alienation.

FORMAL, SYSTEMATIC RESEARCH

Janet Johnston said that alienated children (that is, those who express unreasonable negative feelings and beliefs about a parent) "are likely to be more troubled—more emotionally dependent, less socially competent, have problematic self-esteem (either low or defensively high), poor reality testing, lack the capacity for ambivalence, and are prone to enmeshment or splitting in relations with others" (Johnston, 2005). Johnston and her colleagues collected empirical data that support these clinical observations and reported their findings in an article titled "The psychological functioning of alienated children in custody disputing families: An exploratory study." They analyzed parents' ratings on the Child Behavior Checklist and found that "alienated children had more emotional and behavioral problems of clinically significant proportions compared to their nonalienated counterparts" (Johnston, Walters, and Olesen, 2005a). They administered Rorschach's test to the children and found that "alienated and nonalienated children differ in a number of ways with respect to how they perceive and process information, their preferred coping styles and capacities, and how they express affect."

There has also been systematic, qualitative research regarding the long-term effects of parental alienation on the children (who are sometimes called adult children of parental alienation) as well as on the alienated parents. For example, Amy J. L. Baker (2005a) studied adults who had experienced parental alienation as children. This was a retrospective, qualitative study in which she conducted one-hour, semi-structured interviews of 38 adult children of parental alienation. The transcribed interviews were analyzed for primary themes and patterns. Baker identified several problematic areas in these subjects: high rates of low self-esteem to a point of self-hatred; significant episodes of depression in 70 percent of the subjects; problems with drugs and/or alcohol in about one-third of the subjects; a lack of trust in themselves and in other people; alienation from their own children in 50 percent of the subjects, which suggests that parental alienation is multigenerational; and a high rate of divorce. That is, two-thirds of the participants had been divorced and one-fourth had been divorced more than once, which was higher than the national average. In summarizing this research, the author said, "These findings are not surprising in light of the multiple traumas associated with parental alienation. Not only did the participants experience the loss of a parent but they were also forbidden to mourn that loss or share their thoughts and feelings with their primary caretaker. They were essentially encouraged to deny and/or bury whatever positive regard they had for the targeted parent, cutting off and denying a piece of themselves in the process" (Baker, 2005a).

Baker's book, *Adult Children of Parental Alienation Syndrome: Breaking the Ties That Bind* (Baker, 2007b), explained in greater detail what she learned by interviewing 40 individuals who believed that they had been turned against one parent by the other parent. Baker indicated that her first goal was to determine if people existed who identified themselves as being alienated from one parent due to the behaviors of the other parent. Forty adults were recruited through the Internet or word of mouth, who acknowledged they experienced alienation as a child. According to Baker, the fact that 40 individuals came forward indicates that the concept of parental alienation exists. Of the 40 participants in the study, only 29 indicated their parents divorced during their childhood. In other words, parental alienation can occur in intact families. According to these subjects, the alienating parent was the mother in 34 cases and the father in 6 cases.

Perhaps the most important finding in Baker's study was the identification of three primary patterns of PAS: "(1) narcissistic mothers in divorced families alienating children from the father [14 cases]; (2) narcissistic mothers in intact families alienating the children from the father [10 cases]; and (3) cold, rejecting, or abusive alienating parents of either gender—in intact or divorced families—alienating the children from the targeted parents [16 cases]" (Baker, 2007b, page 14). Based on the data she collected, Baker stated several additional conclusions: many alienating parents seemed to have personality disorders; many alienating parents were also physically or sexually abusive; and alienating parents utilized techniques similar to those used by cult leaders. Baker described 32 parental alienation strategies and concluded that parental alienation is a form of emotional abuse.

In general, Baker's research indicates that the likely long-term effects of parental alienation are: depression due to the lack of ability to mourn and make sense of the loss of the alienated parent; a style of being overly dependent associated with low self-esteem; feelings of guilt when one comes to realize what he or she did to the alienated parent; and difficulties with identity development. The recent research by Baker echoes the observations of John Bowlby in the 1950s. Bowlby said that when the parent-child relationship, the secure base, is destroyed, the consequences are: "Children and adolescents who grow up without their home base providing the necessary support and encouragement are likely to be less cheerful; to find life, especially intimate relationships, difficult; and to be vulnerable in conditions of adversity. In addition, they are likely to have difficulties when they come to marry and have children of their own" (Bowlby, 1988, page 179). With regard to parental alienation, researchers and mental health practitioners have made similar observations and arrived at consistent conclusions, that parental alienation is a form of child abuse and it can leave children with deep, life-long, emotional scars.

17. Parental alienation is a real phenomenon, but controversies related to definitions and terminology have delayed and compromised systematic research regarding this condition. Establishing diagnostic criteria will make it possible to study parental alienation in systematic manner on a larger scale.

There has been a remarkable degree of controversy regarding many aspects of parental alienation since the 1980s. There has been disagreement over what to call this phenomenon: "pathological alignment" (Wallerstein and Kelly, 1976; Johnston, 1993); "visitation refusal" (Wallerstein and Kelly, 1980); "parental alienation syndrome" (Gardner, 1985); "parental alienation" without the word "syndrome" (Garrity and Baris, 1994, page 60); "Medea syndrome" (Wallerstein and Blakeslee, 1989, page 196); "toxic parent" (Cartwright, 1993); "the alienated child" (Kelly and Johnston, 2001, page 251); and "pathological alienation" (Warshak, 2003b).

There has been disagreement over the exact criteria for parental alienation and the causes of this condition. For example, for a child to develop parental alienation, is it necessary for one parent to actively bad-mouth and alienate the child against the second parent? Or, should we say that a child can develop parental alienation as a way to avoid being caught in the crossfire of the parents' battle, even though neither parent actively or purposefully caused the alienation? Can parental alienation be created by social workers who are involved with the family or by the legal process itself?

There has been disagreement over whether parental alienation should be considered a diagnosis, a disorder, a disease, a syndrome, or a "nondiagnostic 'syndrome.'" At times, the debate regarding this topic has been scholarly, esoteric, and adversarial. There has been disagreement as to whether mental health professionals should focus on the continuum of parent-child relationships (with positive relationships at one end and very troubled or alienated relationships at the other) or on the evaluation and treatment of the most severely disturbed youngsters who clearly have parental alienation. The concept of the continuum was developed by Kelly and Johnston (2001), which was meant to demonstrate that there is a variety of responses of children whose parents are separating or divorcing, ranging from normative love and a strong wish to be in close contact with both parents through alignment, realistic estrangement from an abusive parent, and pathological alienation.

Regarding these controversies, "A careful review of the extensive literature indicates that with the exception of two or three writers who reject Gardner's views outright, there is more agreement amongst experienced professionals than there is disagreement" (Fidler et al., 2008a, page 210). There is consensus among almost all mental health professionals who have written about parental alienation regarding the following: (1) Parental alienation is a real entity, that is, there really are children and adolescents who embark on a persistent campaign of denigration against one of the parents and adamantly refuse to see that parent, and the intensity of the campaign and the refusal is far out of proportion to anything the alienated parent has done. (2) There are many causes of contact refusal, and parental alienation is only one of them. (3) Parental alienation is not the correct diagnosis when the child's refusal of contact with a parent is caused by child maltreatment or serious problematic behavior of the alienated parent.

In order for research to be accomplished in a more systematic and comprehensive manner, we need to agree—at least tentatively—on diagnostic criteria. As Turkat (2002) wisely said, "For high quality research to proceed, one must have clear definitions. . . . Without a uniform diagnostic criteria specification, different definitions of PAS could be used which would complicate the interpretation of data across different research studies."

18. Establishing diagnostic criteria will be helpful for: clinicians who work with divorced families; divorced parents, who are trying to do what is best for their children; and children of divorce, who desperately need appropriate treatment that is based on a correct diagnosis.

According to Fidler et al. (2008a), clinical observations, case reviews and qualitative comparative studies uniformly indicate that alienated children may exhibit a variety of symptoms including poor reality testing, illogical cognitive operations, simplistic and rigid information processing, inaccurate or distorted interpersonal perceptions, self-hatred, and other maladaptive attitudes and behaviors. These authors' survey of the short-term and long-term effects of pathological alienation on children reviewed more than 40 articles and chapters published by mental health professionals between 1991 and 2007.

Children with parental alienation should be provided appropriate treatment promptly. Although there may be disagreement about how to conduct the therapy, almost every mental health professional would agree that one goal of treatment is for the child to have a comfortable, healthy, and mutually satisfying relationship with both of his or her parents. The purpose of this book is not to survey all the treatment approaches that have been suggested for parental alienation. Our purpose is to explain why the concept of parental alienation should be included in DSM-5 and ICD-11. However, it is obvious that clinicians need a systematic way to identify and diagnose parental alienation in order for treatment to proceed.

Mild Parental Alienation

If parental alienation is identified early when the symptoms are mild (that is, the child resists contact with the alienated parent, but enjoys his relationship with that parent once parenting time is underway), the treatment can be accomplished by a parenting coordinator who helps the parents communicate in a constructive manner and gives them specific advice regarding their approach to the child's activities with the alienated parent.

A task force of the Association of Family and Conciliation Courts (2006) developed and published a training program for parent coordinators. Michelle Mitcham-Smith, Ph.D., and Wilma J. Henry, Ed.D. (2007), described how parenting coordination may be a helpful inter-

Lack of Treatment Stymies Reunification
Ken Lewis, Ph.D., Philadelphia, Pennsylvania

When she was an infant, Sally's parents divorced. When Sally was 4 years old, her mother was awarded temporary custody and child support at a hearing when the father was not present. That very afternoon, the mother and Sally moved to an unknown location. When Sally was 8 years old, her father's attorney successfully petitioned the court for a custody evaluation and Dr. Lewis was named the evaluator.

Dr. Lewis traced the child support checks to a rural farm in another state and met with Sally and her mother on the farm. Sally, at age 8, was adamant that she never wanted to see her father again because of the horrible things her mother said had been done to them. When Dr. Lewis talked to Sally in private, she reiterated the same complaints that her mother had stated, even using the exact phraseology. Sally said these "bad things" happened two years previously, even though her parents had no contact with each other for the past four years.

When the matter finally came to court, Dr. Lewis was called to testify and offer recommendations. Unfortunately, there was no mental health professional in the county who had any experience with parental alienation and reunification therapy. The court ordered supervised visitation once a month with a social worker, but it never occurred because Sally said she feared her father and refused to go.

vention for parents engaged in high-conflict divorce. Elizabeth M. Ellis, Ph.D., and Susan Boyan, M.Ed., LMFT (in press), also explained specific interventions that parenting coordinators might use to reduce the enmeshment between the alienating parent and the child and strengthen the bond between the targeted parent and the child.

Moderate Parental Alienation

If the parental alienation has reached a moderate degree of severity (the child strongly resists contact and is persistently oppositional during parenting time with the alienated parent), the treatment typically includes more intensive therapy for the child, mother, and father, as well as meetings with the parenting coordinator. If there are multiple therapists involved with the divorced family, they must agree regarding the nature of the problem and the goals of the treatment.

Severe Parental Alienation

If the parental alienation is at a severe degree of intensity (the child adamantly refuses contact and may run away to avoid being with alienated parent), traditional forms of psychotherapy may not be effective. As time goes on, children with parental alienation become intractable in their false beliefs and their mental condition resembles that of individuals with delusional disorder.

Although courts have looked to mental health professionals for recommendations regarding appropriate interventions for severely alienated youngsters, there has been considerable disagreement among the mental health professionals regarding the recommendations. Some mental health professionals have recommended leaving the child with the preferred parent and attempting various combinations of individual and family psychotherapy (e.g., Sullivan and Kelly, 2001). Some mental health professionals have recommended transferring the child from the preferred parent to the custody of the alienated parent (e.g., Gardner, 2001b). Some mental health professionals have recommended doing nothing in circumstances that seem hopeless, allowing the child or adolescent to make his or her own decisions regarding contact with the parents.

Currently, many mental health professionals are taking a more optimistic approach toward the treatment of parental alienation. Douglas Darnall recently published a book regarding the treatment of this condition, *Beyond Divorce Casualties: Reunifying the Alienated Family* (Darnall, 2010). The January 2010 issue of *Family Court Review* was devoted to the treatment of parental alienation. For example, Richard Warshak described a treatment program for children and adolescents with severe parental alienation. The goal of this innovative educational and experiential program—called "Family Bridges"—is to help youngsters repair their damaged relationships with alienated parents in a matter of weeks, not months or years. The program is based on principles such as: focusing on the present and future, not the past; education, not psychotherapy; teaching critical thinking skills, not deprogramming; and saving face and moving on, not requiring apologies for past behaviors. The large majority of children and adolescents who participated in this program achieved and maintained a positive relationship with the previously rejected parent (Warshak, 2010a, 2010b; Warshak and Otis, 2010). In the same issue of *Family Court Review,* another innovative treatment program was described by Sullivan et al. (2010). In their program, called "Overcoming Barriers Family Camp," both parents, significant others, and children participate in a 5-day family camp experience that combines psychoeducation and clinical intervention.

The authors of this book believe that if parental alienation were an official diagnosis, counselors and therapists from all disciplines will become more familiar with this condition. As a result, children with parental alienation will be identified earlier in the course of their illness while it is more easily treated and even cured. Also, if parental alienation were an official diagnosis (with clear criteria for the diagnosis and for severity of the condition), it will be possible to conduct coherent research regarding its treatment.

19. Some mental health professionals have been concerned that if parental alienation were an official diagnosis, the concept would be misused by abusive parents to hide their behavior. On the contrary, establishing diagnostic criteria should *reduce* the opportunities for abusive parents and unethical attorneys to misuse the concept of parental alienation in child custody disputes.

The most common objection to making parental alienation an official diagnosis is that the concept will be misused in legal settings. As Johnston said, "Allegations of [parental alienation syndrome] and [parental alienation] have become a legal strategy in numerous divorce cases when children resist contact with a parent. Largely on the basis of the formulation and recommendations of Gardner, attorneys have vilified the aligned parent and argued for court orders that are coercive and punitive, including a change of custody to the 'hated' other parent in severe cases" (Johnston, 2003).

We agree that in some instances the concept of parental alienation has been misused by abusive parents to hide their behavior. However, we strongly disagree with throwing out the baby with the bathwater. Just because it has been misused does not mean the concept of parental alienation should be denied its place as a recognized diagnosis for mainstream psychology and psychiatry. In fact, the psychiatric diagnosis that is most misused in legal settings is posttraumatic stress disorder. In personal injury lawsuits, the diagnosis of posttraumatic stress disorder in an alleged victim may be used properly or misused by inept evaluators. Also, military veterans and workers' compensation claimants sometimes malinger posttraumatic stress disorder in order to receive disability benefits. However, we are not aware that anybody has proposed that posttraumatic stress disorder should be deleted from DSM because it is sometimes misused.

We believe that the misuse of the concept of parental alienation will be *reduced* rather than increased if parental alienation becomes a diagnosis in DSM and ICD. Having established criteria for the diagnosis of parental alienation will eliminate the babel of conflicting terminology and definitions that currently occurs when parental alienation is mentioned in a legal setting. More important is that the information regarding parental alienation in DSM-5 should include a discussion of the differential diagnosis of contact refusal. It will be clear that the clinician should consider a number of explanations for a child's symptom of contact refusal and not simply rush to the diagnosis of parental alienation. Also, it will be clear that the diagnosis of parental alienation should not be made if the child has a legitimate, justifiable reason for disliking and rejecting one parent, for instance, if the child was neglected or abused by that parent. We believe that when everybody involved in the legal procedures (the parents, the child protection investigators, the mental health professionals, the attorneys, and the judge) has a clear, uniform understanding of the definition of parental alienation, there will be fewer opportunities for rogue expert witnesses and lawyers to misuse the concept in court.

What really matters is whether parental alienation is a real phenomenon, a real entity. If parental alienation is a real clinical entity, it should be included in DSM and ICD. If parental alienation is a real clinical entity, the possibility that the diagnosis may sometimes be misused should not be a primary or serious consideration.

Mother and Therapist Collaborate to Alienate Child
Steve Herman, Ph.D., Hilo, Hawaii

When Tom and Mary divorced, Mary received primary custody of their 3-year-old daughter. After three uneventful post-divorce years of normal visitation and friendly relations, Tom and Mary got into a dispute over the terms of Tom's visitation. Mary initiated legal proceedings to deny Tom normal visitation and voiced suspicions that "something" had happened to their child. A judge selected and appointed an independent psychologist to perform a custody and visitation evaluation. The court-appointed psychologist found no evidence of any abuse by Tom, and described a strong father-daughter relationship. The psychologist recommended normal visitation for Tom.

Unhappy with the opinion of the court-appointed psychologist, Mary spent over $25,000 on at least two different master's level "therapists." The therapists' notes indicate that their sessions focused on trying to get the child to accuse her father of abusing her. According to the notes, the child repeatedly refused to accuse her father of anything worse than making her eat vegetables. She repeatedly told the therapists that she loved her father. After 60 therapy sessions over an eight-month period, the child finally began to make bizarre accusations of sadistic sexual abuse against her father, her father's friends, and other adults. Among other allegations, she accused her father of selling her for prostitution to strangers in hotels during her weekend visitation with him when she was 5 years old.

The sexual abuse accusations led to the complete rupture of the father-daughter relationship and two serious criminal indictments against the father. The indictments against the father were dropped after about three years, when one of the mother's therapists, a key witness in the case, permanently lost his license to practice as a counselor because of fraud and lying to the courts in other disputed custody cases.

Aftermath: Tom has not seen or spoken to his daughter for nine years. Mary continues to pursue the civil case through the courts, seeking, among other things, to have the father reimburse her for $23,000 that she paid the disgraced counselor. The daughter, now 16, says she never wants to see her father again.

20. There are critics of parental alienation and PAS who oppose the use of these concepts as a psychiatric diagnosis, but their arguments are not convincing.

When mental health and legal professionals discuss the prospect that parental alienation will become a diagnosis in DSM-5, the following three concerns are frequently expressed.

(a) There is not enough research for parental alienation to be included in DSM-5. As explained earlier in this book, there is a high threshold for parental alienation or any novel concept to be adopted as a mental disorder in DSM-5. However, the threshold is presumably lower for parental alienation to be included in one of the appendices of DSM-5, that is, Criteria Sets and Axes for Further Study. The threshold is definitely lower for parental alienation to be considered one of the relational problems, which are currently included in the chapter in DSM-IV-TR called Other Conditions That May Be a Focus of Clinical Attention. The professional papers, book chapters, and books discussed in this proposal and listed in the bibliography clearly prove that parental alienation exists and affects hundreds of thousands of children and their families. There clearly is enough qualitative and quantitative research for parental alienation to be included among the criteria sets for further study or the relational problems, if not for full inclusion as a mental disorder in DSM-5.

The magnitude of research that has been accomplished to date is evidence that parental alienation and PAS are already established as working mental health diagnoses. Including parental alienation in DSM-5 will reflect a reality that already exists. Once parental alienation is included in DSM-5, the universal ability to rely on clear definitions and consistent diagnostic criteria will help ensure the highest levels of replicability and accuracy across individual researchers and across cultures.

(b) If parental alienation becomes a diagnosis in DSM-5, it will be misused in court by abusive parents to take their children away from protective parents. This is sometimes called the "Henry Ford argument," that is, "Henry Ford should not have invented the automobile assembly line because so many people are injured and killed in motor vehicle accidents." The authors of this proposal obviously do not condone the misuse of the concepts of parental alienation or PAS. We believe that the morbidity due to parental alienation is much, much greater than that caused by the occasional misuse of the concept. We realize that divorc-

ing parents sometimes accuse each other of causing parental alien-ation, but we believe it is rare that these accusations actually result in an abusive parent's gaining custody of his or her children. We predict that when parental alienation is clearly defined and the concept is cor-rectly understood–including the provision that it does not pertain when the rejected parent has been abusive or neglectful–there will be less opportunity for abusive parents and unscrupulous attorneys to misuse the concept.

(c) The notion of parental alienation puts too much blame on the parent who is accused of causing the alienation. There has been confusion between Richard Gardner's concept of PAS and the definition of parental alien-ation as proposed in this document. Gardner's concept of PAS includ-ed the idea that one of the parents actively influenced the child to fear and despise the other parent. Although we believe that occurs in many instances, it is not necessary to have an alienating parent for parental alienation to occur. Parental alienation may occur simply in the con-text of a high-conflict divorce in which the parents fight and the child aligns with one side to get out of the middle of the battle, even with no indoctrination by the favored parent. Parental alienation may be brought about by extended family members, social service personnel involved with the family, or the adversarial nature of the legal system. Our definition of parental alienation is that a child gravitates to one parent (the preferred parent) and refuses contact with the other parent (the alienated parent) without legitimate justification. In our definition, we do not even use the term, "alienating parent," but refer to the "pre-ferred parent." Our suggested criteria for parental alienation disorder in Appendix A and parental alienation relational problem in App-endix B focus on the behaviors and symptoms of the child, not on the behavior of the preferred parent.

There have been several highly publicized articles in the profes-sional literature that criticize Gardner's concept of PAS. These articles have little direct impact on this proposal because they primarily per-tain to PAS, not on parental alienation as defined in this book. Also, these authors challenged specific statements in Gardner's writings or simply raised *ad hominem* attacks on Gardner himself. Since Gardner first used the term "parental alienation syndrome" in 1985, hundreds of mental health and legal professionals have researched, studied, and commented on the phenomenon of parental alienation. There is no need now to dwell on the details of what Richard Gardner did or said or wrote. In the interests of completeness, however, we summarize the following critiques of Gardner and PAS, which are in chronological order. Readers who desire more information regarding these controversies may want to read "Bringing Sense to Parental Alienation: A Look at the Disputes and the Evidence" (Warshak, 2003a); "L'aliénation parentale: Points controversés" ("Parental Alienation: Controversies") (French) (Van Gijseghem, 2005a); "Parental Alienation Syndrome: Detractors and the Junk Science Vacuum" (Lorandos, 2006a); and "The Spectrum of Parental Alienation Syndrome (Part IV): Critics of Parental Alienation Syndrome and the Politics of Science" (Rand, in press).

Cheri L. Wood

Cheri Wood (1994), a law student, published a law review article, "The Parental Alienation Syndrome: A Dangerous Aura of Reliability." She wrote that Richard Gardner's definition of PAS was used primarily for the purpose of invalidating charges of sexual abuse in courts of law. Wood was mistaken in asserting that PAS was centered upon sexual abuse or Gardner's Sexual Abuse Legitimacy scale—in fact, the eight manifestations of PAS identified by Gardner do not include allegations of sexual abuse at all. Wood made two major points in her article. In the section, "Causation Problems with PAS," she explained that for a determination that PAS was present, it would have to be shown that the alienation was actually caused by the alienating parent and not by other factors such as psychological, social, and legal-system stressors. In the section, "Evidentiary Problems with PAS," Wood explained in detail the *Frye* and *Daubert* tests for admissibility of scientific evidence. Wood concluded that under either of these tests, testimony regarding PAS should not be accepted because, "Dr. Gardner based his theory entirely upon his own observations of his own patients; it is for the most part self-published, which circumvents peer review; and it has attracted anything but widespread acceptance." Wood claimed that at the time of her writing, the greater professional community did not accept PAS, as if scholars were a single unit with no deviating theoretical frameworks. Since Ms. Wood published that article, hundreds of articles and book chapters from many countries have discussed parental alienation and PAS, so perhaps her concern about their acceptance in the scientific community has been resolved.

Danielle Isman

Danielle Isman (1996), apparently a law student at the University of California, Davis, published a law review article, "Gardner's Witch-hunt." Isman persistently misrepresented Gardner's writings, and then criticized those misrepresentations. In her opening paragraphs, for example, Isman said, "Gardner believes that whenever a child expresses dislike of or apprehension about contact with the father, and the mother is the primary caretaker, the reason for the child's reservations about the father are caused by the mother's abuse." Also, "According to Gardner, any time a child has an extreme dislike of his or her father, the mother caused the animosity." Most readers of this book will immediately understand that Richard Gardner did not express either of those opinions.

Kathleen C. Faller, Ph.D.

Kathleen Faller (1998), a professor of social work at the University of Michigan, published "The Parental Alienation Syndrome: What Is It and What Data Support it?" In that article, Faller extensively criticized Gardner and his writings regarding PAS, especially his statistics. Faller criticized Gardner for overestimating the frequency of false allegations of sexual abuse in disputed custody cases, but she agreed that false allegations sometimes do occur in these cases. Faller criticized Gardner for overestimating the percentage of false allegations of abuse made by mothers, but she seemed to agree that both mothers and fathers sometimes make false allegations. In her conclusions, Faller said that PAS should not be used to determine whether or not the child was actually abused by one of the parents, e.g., the father. She said, "Its only possible utility may be in understanding the behavior of the child and mother in some cases in which the allegation of mistreatment by the father is determined by other means to be false." Of course, that is what most writers have said all along regarding PAS, that the concept only applies when it is known that the child's reluctance to see the rejected parent is not based on maltreatment by that parent. Faller's article was discussed and critiqued by Gardner (1998d).

Carol S. Bruch, J.D.

Carol Bruch (2001a, 2001b, and 2002) a law professor, published substantially the same law review article, "Parental Alienation Syn-drome and Parental Alienation: Getting it Wrong in Child Custody Cases," in three journals. Bruch misstated the central hypothesis of Gardner's "theory" regarding PAS; she asserted that Gardner coined the term to describe cases that he felt involved false allegations of sex-ual abuse. Bruch put much energy into criticizing Gardner's published writings such as: Gardner's estimates of the prevalence of PAS; his emphasis on the possibility that the child is lying about being abused; his recommended treatment for serious cases; and his belief that PAS sometimes constitutes *folie à deux*. Bruch put much energy into criti-cizing Gardner himself: the exact nature of his faculty appointment at Columbia University; he self-published some of his works; he had a personal website; Gardner's website had links from the websites of fathers' organizations; and Gardner referenced his own publications in subsequent publications. Bruch was alarmed that, "The media, par-ents, therapists, lawyers, mediators, and judges now often refer to PAS, many apparently assuming that it is a scientifically established and useful mental health diagnosis" (Bruch, 2001b). Regarding the future, Bruch said, "The first question is whether scientific sufficiency has been indicated by respected professional vetting, for example, inclu-sion in the American Psychiatric Association's DSM-IV or the World Health Organization's ICD-10" (Bruch, 2001b). We agree with Professor Bruch that the inclusion of parental alienation in these books will help clarify a good deal of the confusion regarding this concept. Bruch's article was comprehensively discussed and critiqued by Gardner (see *www.pas-konferenz.de/e/dok/garnderbruch_e. doc*).

Jennifer Hoult, J.D.

Jennifer Hoult (2006), an attorney, offered an extensive literature review, claiming to analyze every precedent-bearing court decision and every law review referencing PAS published in the previous twen-ty years. In appendices, Hoult listed 64 precedent-bearing U.S. cases that referenced PAS; she listed 112 law review articles that referenced PAS. Hoult concluded that PAS, at least in Gardner's original formu-lation, should be inadmissible in court because it is a mere *ipse dixit*, a form of "pseudo-science" that fails to meet general legal requirements for admissibility into evidence. Hoult identified recognized challenges in the diagnosis of alienation, such as difficulties in distinguishing justified from unjustified alienation, the difficulty of proving causation, and the paucity of empirical data on diagnostic reliability. Hoult implicitly addressed the importance of subjecting parental alienation to the scrutiny of the DSM-5 Task Force, noting, "Designation as a medical syndrome, as represented by inclusion in the *Diagnostic and Statistical Manual of Mental Disorders* (DSM), represents a proxy for scientific verification." Hoult also accurately identified elements of the PAS literature whose value is called into question by high levels of self-citation. However, many other criticisms were painted with a very broad brush that failed to differentiate issues with the concept of PAS from matters of poor professional practice that would be unacceptable regardless of what diagnostic categories were at issue. For example, Hoult complained that the concept of PAS has been used to diagnose the behavior of mothers when only their children have been examined. At times, Hoult became so enthusiastic in criticizing Gardner's writings that she slipped into hyperbole, referring, for instance, to "PAS's presumption that abuse allegations are always false" and stating that, according to Gardner, "[Incest] can never be the basis for justified alienation," and that, "[PAS] presumes all reports of male violence are false" (Hoult, 2006). To our knowledge, these characterizations of PAS and Gardner's opinions are totally mistaken. However, based on these mistaken opinions, Hoult concluded that "PAS is, and should remain, inadmissible in American courts" (Hoult, 2006).

Two national organizations of legal professionals have criticized the use of parental alienation and PAS in legal proceedings. As far as we can tell, the authors of the following "judge's guides" do not base their opinions on Gardner's own articles and books or the vast international literature regarding these topics, but on the ambiguous statement by the American Psychological Association (2008) and the writings of Faller (1998), Bruch (2001a, 2001b, and 2002), and Hoult (2006).

National Council of Juvenile and Family Court Judges (NCJFCJ)

In 2004 and again in 2006, the NCJFCJ released a document, "Navigating Custody & Visitation Evaluations in Cases with Domestic Violence: A Judge's Guide." The authors of the JCJFCJ document stated, "In contested custody cases, children may indeed express fear of, be concerned about, have distaste for, or be angry at one of their parents. Unfortunately, an all too common practice in such cases is for evaluators to diagnose children who exhibit a very strong bond and alignment with one parent and, simultaneously, a strong rejection of the other parent, as suffering from 'parental alienation syndrome' or 'PAS.' Under relevant evidentiary standards, the court should not accept this testimony" (NCJFCJ, 2006, page 24). A footnote to this passage states, "'Parental alienation syndrome' was introduced by Richard Gardner and was primarily associated with child sexual abuse allegations in the context of contested child custody cases. For more information, see Bruch, supra note 28." In the NCJDCJ document, footnote 28 said, "We refer to cases in which the children may express fear of, be concerned about, have distaste for, or be angry at one of their parents as being estranged from the parent. We do not use the labels of 'parental alienation,' 'alienation,' or 'parental alienation syndrome' to describe this behavior because to do so would give credibility to a 'theory' that has been discredited by the scientific community" (NCJFCJ, 2006, page 14).

In support of this sweeping rejection of the concept of parental alienation, the authors of the NCJFCJ document cited exactly three sources: the statement by the American Psychological Association (1996), which was discussed on page 99 of this book, and the articles by Faller (1998) and Bruch (2002), which were discussed above. When the authors of the NCJFCJ document stated that parental alienation has been "discredited," they apparently were not aware of the hundreds of articles, book chapters, and books that are discussed in this book and listed in the bibliography.

American Bar Association (ABA)

In 2008, two components of the ABA—the Child Custody and Adoption Pro Bono Project and the Center on Children and the Law—released the second edition of a lengthy handbook, *A Judge's Guide: Making Child-Centered Decisions in Custody Cases.* The authors of the ABA document stated, "Related to the Friendly Parent Provision is the controversial issue of Parental Alienation Syndrome. Under this theory, a parent who 'bad mouths' another parent in front of the child, or 'brain washes' the child to turn against the other parent, is considered to be not acting in the child's best interests. This theory is highly controversial and has largely been discredited as bad science" (ABA, 2008, page 134). A footnote to this passage simply cites the article by

Bruch (2001b). The bibliography for that section also cited the article by Hoult (2006).

The authors of the ABA document also stated, "For psychologists without training in the dynamics of domestic violence, the abused parent's efforts to protect herself and her children could easily be misinterpreted as intentionally alienating the batterer-parent. This in spite of the American Psychological Associations' determination that there exists no scientific basis for the theory of parental alienation syndrome" (ABA, 2008, page 251). A footnote suggests that the authors of the ABA document were referring to the statement by the American Psychological Association (1996). When the authors of the ABA book said that PAS "has largely been discredited" and that "there exists no scientific basis" for PAS, they apparently were not aware of the hundreds of articles, book chapters, and books that are discussed in this book and listed in the bibliography.

National District Attorneys Association (NDAA)

Some critics have stated that the NDAA has rejected parental alienation or PAS. Actually, the NDAA has no opinion regarding these topics. The critics of parental alienation are probably referring to a two-part article that was published in the newsletter of NDAA. Erika Rivera Ragland and Hope Fields—not NDAA itself—expressed the opinion, "At best, PAS is a nondiagnostic 'syndrome' that only explains the behavior of the child and the mother when there is a known false allegation [of domestic violence]. It is a courtroom diagnosis befitting adversaries involved in legal sparring. It is not capable of lending itself to hard data or inclusion in the forthcoming DSM-V" (Ragland and Fields, 2003). The purpose of that article was to guide child abuse prosecutors in understanding and challenging the theory of PAS if it is presented in court.

Janet R. Johnston, Ph.D., and Joan B. Kelly, Ph.D.

While this proposal was being developed, early versions were widely distributed among psychologists, psychiatrists, and other interested parties. Shortly before this manuscript was sent to the publisher, Janet Johnston and Joan Kelly sent a letter to DSM-5 personnel objecting to our proposal that parental alienation be included in DSM-5 (personal communication, Janet Johnston, 2009).

We agree with some of the observations of Johnston and Kelly. For example, we agree that our estimate of the prevalence of parental alienation (in Section 12, page 96) is a very rough estimate. They say, "Wide variations in definition and measurement produce invalid estimates," which is exactly why parental alienation needs to be formally defined in DSM-5. Of course, there are serious debates regarding the prevalence of childhood conditions that are already in DSM–bipolar disorder, for example.

We agree with Johnston and Kelly that the words "parental alienation" have been used in the professional literature to mean different concepts and behaviors. We all know that is a problem and in this document we carefully defined what we mean by "parental alienation." The extensive confusion regarding terminology that concerns Johnston and Kelly is, of course, a good reason to define "parental alienation" in DSM-5 so future clinicians and researchers will use the words in a consistent manner.

We agree with Johnston and Kelly that sometimes it is hard to distinguish parental alienation from "realistic estrangement due to problematic or abusive parenting." Of course, it is necessary to rule out child abuse by the rejected parent before making the diagnosis of parental alienation. However, the evaluator has the very same problem when making the diagnosis of sexual abuse of a child, since one must assess whether the alleged abuse really happened or was fabricated. The evaluator has the same problem in making the diagnosis of delusional disorder, since one must assess whether the patient's beliefs, which are not bizarre, are true or false.

We agree with Johnston and Kelly when they say, "The research on the etiology of the disorder/problem is largely exploratory in nature and needs to be further developed." That is true but irrelevant. In fact, there are many conditions in DSM for which the etiology is not known–autistic disorder, for example. For a condition to be included in DSM, it is not necessary to know its etiology.

We agree with Johnston and Kelly that "there is currently heated dialogue and controversy amongst professionals in the forensic family law field with response to treatment of parental alienation." That is true but irrelevant. There are many conditions in DSM for which there is debate regarding treatment or there is no satisfactory treatment. For a condition to be included in DSM, it is not necessary for it to be treatable.

Finally, we agree with Johnston and Kelly that no one knows at this time exactly what all the criteria should be for the diagnosis of parental alienation. The criteria that we propose are based on many articles and book chapters in the professional literature regarding parental alienation, and they make sense in both theoretical and empirical terms. Clinicians all over the world are already "diagnosing" parental alienation using whatever fragmented, disorganized criteria they can get their hands on. We will be doing these clinicians a great service by taking the information that is currently available, coming up with the best set of definitions and criteria we can, and presenting it to them through DSM-5. Of course, once a diagnosis is in DSM, the criteria may be adjusted in future editions.

Rather than continue to write rebuttals—which are then followed by rebuttals to the rebuttals—we hope that mental health and legal professionals who are concerned about the children of divorced parents come together to find common ground. We all seem to agree regarding core issues, that parental alienation is a serious problem that causes considerable morbidity for many thousands of children and their families. We need to call a truce to the feuding that has occurred among the scholars and clinicians who have written about this topic. We need to agree—at a minimum—on definitions and terminology. The development of DSM-5 is a wonderful opportunity to achieve that goal. Once we have agreed on terminology and criteria for the diagnosis, there will be plenty of time in the future to do additional research regarding diagnostic precision, differential diagnosis, etiology, treatment, and prognosis.

Chapter Three

PUBLISHED CRITERIA FOR A
NEW DIAGNOSIS IN DSM-5

In about November 2009 (after most of this book was written), DSM-5 Task Force personnel posted on their website an important document, "Guidelines for Making Changes to DSM-V" (Kendler et al., 2009). Although the principles in this document were not intended to be construed as inflexible or unalterable rules, they do provide important guidance for the various work groups that will make decisions regarding DSM-5. Since we have already discussed in detail "Twenty Reasons Why Parental Alienation Should be a Diagnosis," it is not difficult to apply the data in this book to the recently published criteria for a new diagnosis in DSM-5. There are no references in this chapter to primary source material, but we refer the reader to the sections of this book where each topic is discussed. In the following text, the criteria suggested by Kendler et al. are in bold font.

The Guidelines state that **a proposal for change in the current diagnostic classification should be supported by an explication of the *reasons* for the proposed change**. Parental alienation should be adopted as a psychiatric diagnosis because: (1) Parental alienation consists of a mental component, i.e., the child's firmly held false belief that the alienated parent is an evil, dangerous, or worthless person. (2) As a result of the false belief, the child manifests seriously maladaptive behavior, i.e., refusal to have contact with the alienated parent. (3) Parental alienation causes considerable morbidity, i.e., the loss of the child's relationship with a loving parent and numerous other symptoms (pages 110 to 119). (4) Hundreds of thousands of children are affected by this condition (pages 96 to 98).

The proposal should include **a discussion of possible unintended negative effects of this proposed change, if it is made, and a consideration of arguments against making this change**. Some writers have expressed the concern that it is hard to tell the difference between parental alienation (when the child's refusal to see the rejected parent is unjustified) and parental estrangement (when the child's refusal to see the rejected parent is realistic). Of course, that is the whole point of this proposal, that it is essential for clinicians and forensic evaluators to do the best they can at making that distinction. A proper assessment is necessary for parental alienation as it is for any diagnostic category in DSM-5. A professional needs to consider the differential diagnosis. There are negative consequences of any diagnosis when the evaluation is done by a person who is inexperienced or unqualified.

Some writers have expressed the concern that judges may mistakenly rely on the concept of parental alienation to transfer custody of a child from a protective parent to an abusive parent. However, we conclude that the known positive effects of the proposed new diagnosis are much, much greater than the unlikely and speculative negative effects. The arguments that have been raised against the adoption of parental alienation as a DSM-5 diagnosis are discussed on pages 127 to 136.

Adding a new diagnosis to DSM-5 constitutes a major change, so there should be considerable support for the validity of the proposed diagnosis. Kendler et al. suggested the following guidelines for assessing this issue, starting with:

(1) **A broad consensus of expert clinical opinion would generally be expected for all proposed changes or additions to DSM-5**. The 70 contributing authors of this proposal include psychiatrists and psychologists from twelve countries. We have explained how parental alienation was discovered independently by six researchers or research teams in the 1980s, and it has been described in at least 30 countries throughout the world (pages 52 to 80). The bibliography of this book contains hundreds of scientific papers, book chapters, and books from the professional literature (pages 187 to 230). There is no doubt among mental health professionals who evaluate and treat children of divorce that the phenomenon of parental alienation occurs and causes considerable suffering and impairment.

(2) **In most situations, we would expect modest changes to have at least some support from the validators listed above**.

(3) **Substantial and especially major changes should generally have broad support from several validator classes and particularly from at least one high priority validator. For most major changes, we would expect to see support from several high priority validators**. The addition of a new diagnosis is a "major change." There is an enormous amount of qualitative research and a limited amount of quantitative research regarding parental alienation. The validators listed in the Guidelines are organized in the following manner:

3a. Antecedent Validators, such as: familial aggregation; sociodemographic and cultural factors; environmental risk factors; and prior psychiatric history. With regard to parental alienation, this mental condition is characterized by familial aggregation, that is, in most cases multiple siblings are affected. Also, it is obvious that environmental risk factors play a role, since parental alienation almost always occurs in the context of a high-conflict divorce.

3b. Concurrent Validators, such as: cognitive, emotional, temperament, and personality correlates (unrelated to the diagnostic criteria); biological markers; and patterns of comorbidity. Of course, we would not expect to find biological markers of parental alienation since it is clearly caused by environmental factors and life experiences. However, parental alienation does manifest comorbidity in the sense of a collection of symptoms that frequently occur together. The typical symptoms are noted in Appendix A of this book and personality correlates were discussed in Section 16 (pages 110 to 119).

3c. Predictive Validators, such as: diagnostic stability; course of illness; and response to treatment. In terms of qualitative research, there have been many reports that the diagnostic stability depends on the severity of the condition. Mild parental alienation typically resolves spontaneously. Moderately severe parental alienation may continue through adolescence. However, severe parental alienation frequently continues unabated, clearly into adulthood, unless some form of intervention occurs (pages 110 to 119).

(4) **Substantial and especially major changes should rarely if ever be based solely on reports from a single researcher or research team**. This criterion is hardly a problem with regard to

parental alienation. Six researchers or research teams independently described parental alienation in the 1980s (pages 24 to 32). Using the criteria specified in these initial publications, scores of authors identified children with parental alienation in their own research subjects and clinical practices (pages 32 to 80).

(5) **Major changes should generally require consistency of support across validators. In particular, we would not generally expect to support substantial and especially major changes if a significant proportion of the literature contained evidence that contradicted the change (i.e., statistically significant results in the wrong direction).** We are not aware of any publication in the literature of psychiatry, psychology, or social work that concludes that parental alienation–as the concept is defined in this book–does not exist.

(6) **Generally, for substantial and particularly major changes, at least some of the supporting literature should be of high methodologic quality.** Regarding the validity of the concept of parental alienation, there is an enormous amount of qualitative research, much of it conducted by highly qualified and well-known authors (pages 24 to 42). Regarding the reliability of the diagnostic criteria and the prevalence of parental alienation, there is a modest amount of quantitative research (pages 91 to 98). We conclude that it is clear that parental alienation exists; scores of experienced clinicians have identified parental alienation in thousands of children. We conclude that some degree of parental alienation–whether mild, moderate or severe–occurs in approximately 1 percent of children in the U.S. Once the definition and the diagnostic criteria for parental alienation are established, it will be possible to conduct more extensive research to test the reliability of those criteria.

Kendler et al. (2009) also suggested the following "additional considerations for evaluatting proposed new diagnoses to be included in DSM-V":

(1) **A need for the category–Here the key question is whether the proposed category identifies a distinct group of people who need appropriate clinical attention.** We believe that parental alienation is a treatable condition when it is identified in the early stages, that is, mild and moderate degrees of severity. This condition is very difficult and expensive to treat when it becomes severe (pages 121 to

124). Once parental alienation is accepted as a diagnostic entity, both trainees and practicing clinicians will learn about it, identify it, and treat parental alienation before it becomes chronic and intractable.

(2) **Relationship with other DSM-5 diagnoses–Here the key question is whether the diagnosis is sufficiently distinct from other diagnoses to warrant being considered a separate diagnosis**. An inexperienced clinician might confuse parental alienation with the following conditions: separation anxiety disorder (because the child is afraid to leave the side of the preferred parent); oppositional defiant disorder (because the child refuses to follow the requests of the alienated parent); and shared psychotic disorder (because both the preferred parent and the child appear delusional that the alienated parent is evil, dangerous, or worthless). These and other possibilities are discussed in the section regarding differential diagnosis in Appendix A of this book (pages 147 to 151). Although parental alienation may superficially look like separation anxiety disorder or oppositional defiant disorder, they are obviously distinct disorders because they have different etiologies: parental alienation usually occurs in the context of a high-conflict divorce and frequently involves one parent who is consciously or unconsciously indoctrinating the child against the other parent. Also, it is very important to distinguish parental alienation from these other conditions because the treatment is different.

(3) **Potential harm–Is there potential for harm to affected individuals or other groups of persons because of the adoption of this category in DSM-5? Could the harm that arises from the adoption of the proposed diagnosis exceed the benefit that would accrue to affected individuals?** This topic was already addressed in the discussion of "possible unintended negative effects of this proposed change." Also, see pages 127 to 136.

(4) **Available treatments–Is there evidence that, if the diagnosis were included in DSM-5, that any effective biological, psychological, or social treatments for this diagnosis could potentially be found?** There have been journal articles, chapters, books, and professional conferences devoted to the treatment of parental alienation (pages 121 to 124).

(5) **Meets criteria for a mental (psychiatric) diagnosis. Finally, any proposed set of criteria for a category to be included in**

DSM-5 should identify a mental or psychiatric diagnosis and not variations of normal psychological functioning. It is common for children of divorce parents to develop loyalty conflicts. That is, these children have affection for both parents and it is upsetting for them to see their parents argue and, ultimately, separate and divorce. To some extent, the set of children with severe loyalty conflicts will overlap with the set of children with a mild degree of parental alienation. It is reasonable to conclude that some children with subclinical or mild parental alienation are simply manifesting a more or less normal reaction to their parents' divorce. However, children with moderate and severe forms of parental alienation are certainly not manifesting normal psychological functioning. It is simply not normal for a child to develop a firmly held, false belief that one of his parents is evil, dangerous, or worthless and–based on that false belief–adamantly refuse to have contact with that parent, thus losing a most important relationship for many years and perhaps a lifetime. Children with moderate and severe parental alienation develop a wide variety of secondary symptoms including anxiety, depression, suicidality, dependency issues, intimacy issues, fears of abandonment, and impaired cognitive skills (pages 110 to 119).

We believe that we have adequately demonstrated that parental alienation–as defined in this proposal–meets the criteria for a new diagnosis in DSM-5 stated by Kendler et al. (2009). If DSM-5 personnel conclude there is not enough systematic research for parental alienation disorder to be in the main text of DSM-5, there is undoubtedly enough evidence for it to be placed in the appendix, Criteria Sets and Axes for Further Study. As we explained at the beginning of this book, parental alienation can be conceptualized as either a "mental disorder" or a "relational problem." It is possible that DSM-5 personnel will conclude that this mental condition should be classified as parental alienation relational problem and included in the chapter of DSM-5, "Other Conditions That May Be a Focus of Clinical Attention."

Chapter Four

CONCLUSIONS AND RECOMMENDATIONS

Parental alienation affects hundreds of thousands of children in the U.S. and comparable numbers around the world. Parental alienation has been recognized by thousands of mental health and legal professionals. It is treated by thousands of psychologists, psychiatrists, social workers, and family counselors. There is no doubt that parental alienation is recognized by the vast majority of mental health professionals who work with children of divorced parents. There is no doubt it is a real diagnostic entity. We agree that in some instances the concept of parental alienation has been misused by abusive parents and unscrupulous attorneys. There should be additional research on this topic, and diagnostic criteria need to be established so that more systematic research can be undertaken and its misuse can be prevented.

We recommend that diagnostic criteria for parental alienation disorder be included in DSM-5 and ICD-11. With regard to DSM-5, we propose that the text in Appendix A (regarding parental alienation disorder) be included in the part of the book regarding mental disorders *or* the text in Appendix B (regarding parental alienation relational problem) be included in the discussion of relational problems. With regard to ICD-11, we propose that the text in Appendix A (regarding parental alienation disorder) should be included in the section of Chapter V called "Behavioural and emotional disorders with onset usually occurring in childhood and adolescence" or the text in Appendix B (regarding parental alienation relational problem) should be included in the section of Chapter XXI called "Problems related to negative life events in childhood." Parental alienation disorder should be recognized as a serious condition that affects many children and families throughout the world.

Readers who wish to express their opinions regarding this topic to DSM-5 personnel may send written materials to the following:

> David J. Kupfer, M.D.
> (Chair of the DSM-5 Task Force)
> Director of Research
> Western Psychiatric Institute and Clinic
> 3811 O'Hara Street
> Pittsburgh, PA 15213

> Darrel A. Regier, M.D.
> (Vice-chair of the DSM-5 Task Force)
> Director, APA Division of Research
> American Psychiatric Association
> 1000 Wilson Blvd., Suite 1825
> Arlington, VA 22209–3901

> Daniel S. Pine, M.D.
> (Chair of the DSM-5 Disorders in Childhood and Adolescence Work Group)
> Chief, Section on Development and Affective Neuroscience
> National Institutes of Mental Health
> 15K North Drive, MSC-2670
> Bethesda, MD 20892–2670

Readers who wish to express their opinions regarding this topic to ICD-11 personnel may send written materials to the following:

> Geoffrey M. Reed, Ph.D.
> Department of Mental Health and Substance Abuse
> (MSD/MER)
> World Health Organization
> 20, Avenue Appia
> CH-1211 Geneva 27
> Switzerland

APPENDICES

Appendix A

PROPOSED CRITERIA FOR
PARENTAL ALIENATION DISORDER

DIAGNOSTIC FEATURES

The essential feature of **parental alienation disorder** is that a child—usually one whose parents are engaged in a high-conflict divorce—allies himself or herself strongly with one parent (the preferred parent) and rejects a relationship with the other parent (the alienated parent) without legitimate justification. The primary behavioral symptom is the child's resistance or refusal to have contact with the alienated parent (Criterion A).

The behaviors in the child that characterize **parental alienation disorder** include a persistent campaign of denigration against the alienated parent and weak, frivolous, and absurd rationalizations for the child's criticism of the alienated parent (Criterion B).

The following clinical features frequently occur in **parental alienation disorder**, especially when the child's symptoms reach a level that is moderate or severe (Criterion C). Lack of ambivalence refers to the child's belief that the alienated parent is all bad and the preferred parent is all good. The independent-thinker phenomenon means that the child proudly states the decision to reject the alienated parent is his own, not influenced by the preferred parent. Reflexive support of the preferred parent against the alienated parent refers to the pattern of the child's immediately and automatically taking the preferred parent's side in a disagreement. The child may exhibit a disregard for the feelings of the alienated parent and an absence of guilt over exploitation of the alienated parent. The child may manifest borrowed scenarios, that is, rehearsed statements that are identical to those made by the preferred parent. Also, the child's animosity toward the alienated parent may spread to that parent's extended family.

The diagnosis of **parental alienation disorder** should not be used if the child's refusal to have contact with the rejected parent is justifiable, for example, if the child was neglected or abused by that parent (Criterion D).

ASSOCIATED FEATURES

Parental alienation disorder may be mild, moderate, or severe. When the **parental alienation disorder** is mild, the child may briefly resist contact with the alienated parent, but does have contact and enjoys a good relationship with the alienated parent once they are together. When the **parental alienation disorder** is mild, the child may have a strong, healthy relationship with both parents, even though the child recites criticisms of the alienated parent.

When the **parental alienation disorder** is moderate, the child may persistently resist contact with the alienated parent and will continue to complain and criticize the alienated parent during the contact. The child is likely to have a mildly to moderately pathological relationship with the preferred parent.

When the **parental alienation disorder** is severe, the child strongly and persistently resists contact and may hide or run away to avoid seeing the alienated parent. The child's behavior is driven by a firmly-held, false belief that the alienated parent is evil, dangerous, or worthless. The child is likely to have a strong, severely pathological relationship with the preferred parent, perhaps sharing a paranoid world view.

While the diagnosis of **parental alienation disorder** refers to the child, the preferred parent and other persons the child is dependent on may manifest the following attitudes and behaviors, which frequently are the major cause of the disorder: persistent criticisms of the rejected parent's personal qualities and parenting activities; statements that influence the child to fear, dislike, and criticize the alienated parent; and various maneuvers to exclude the rejected parent from the child's life. The behavior of the preferred parent may include complaints to the police and child protection agencies with allegations about the rejected parent. **Parental alienation disorder** may be the basis for false allegations of sexual abuse against the alienated parent. The preferred parent may be litigious to the point of abusing the legal system. The preferred parent may violate court orders that are not to his or her liking. Specific psychological problems—narcissistic personality disorder, borderline personality disorder, traumatic childhood experiences, and paranoid traits—may be identified in these individuals.

Also, the rejected parent may manifest the following attitudes and behaviors, which may be a minor or contributory cause of the disorder: lack of warm, involved parenting; deficient parenting skills; and lack of time dedicated to parenting activities. However, the intensity and duration of the child's refusal to have contact with the rejected parent is far out of proportion to the relatively minor weaknesses in the rejected parent's parenting skills.

Although **parental alienation disorder** most often arises in the context of a child-custody dispute between two parents, it can arise in other types of conflicts over child custody, such as a dispute between a parent and stepparent or between a parent and a grandparent. Sometimes, other family members–such as stepparents or grandparents–contribute to the creation of **parental alienation disorder**. On occasion, other individuals–such as therapists and child protection workers–contribute to the creation of **parental alienation disorder** by encouraging or supporting the child's refusal to have contact with the alienated parent. Also, **parental alienation disorder** does not necessarily appear in the context of divorce litigation, but may occur in intact families or years following the divorce.

DIFFERENTIAL DIAGNOSIS

It is common for children to resist or avoid contact with the noncustodial parent after the parents separate or divorce. There are several possible explanations for a child's active rejection of contact. **Parental alienation disorder** is an important, but not the only, reason that children refuse contact.

In the course of normal development children will become polarized with one parent and then the other depending on the child's developmental stage and events in the child's life. When parents disagree, it is normal for children to experience loyalty conflicts. These transitory variations in a child's relationship with his or her parents do not meet criteria for **parental alienation disorder** because they do not constitute "a persistent rejection or denigration of a parent that reaches the level of a campaign."

If the child actually was abused, neglected, or disliked by the noncustodial parent or the current boyfriend or girlfriend of that parent, the child's animosity may be justified and it is understandable that the child would not want to visit the rejected parent's household. If abuse were the reason for the child's refusal, the diagnosis would be **physical abuse of child** or **sexual abuse of child**, not **parental alienation disorder**. This is important to keep in mind because an abusive, rejected parent may misuse the concept of **parental alienation disorder** in order to falsely blame the child's refusal of contact on the parent that the child prefers.

In **shared psychotic disorder**, a delusional parent may influence a child to believe that the other parent is an evil person who must be feared and avoided. In **parental alienation disorder**, the alienating parent may have very strong opinions about the alienated parent, but is not usually considered out of touch with reality.

When parents separate or divorce, a child with **separation anxiety disorder** may become even more worried and anxious about being away from the primary caretaker. In **separation anxiety disorder**, the child is preoccupied with unrealistic fears that something will happen to the primary caretaker, while the child with **parental alienation disorder** is preoccupied with unrealistic beliefs that the alienated parent is dangerous.

It is conceivable that a child with **specific phobia, situational type**, might have an unreasonable fear of a parent or some aspect of the parent's household. A child with a **specific phobia** is unlikely to engage in a persistent campaign of denigration against the feared object, while the campaign of denigration is a central feature of **parental alienation disorder**.

When parents separate or divorce, a child with **oppositional defiant disorder** may become even more symptomatic—angry, resentful, stubborn—and not want to participate in the process of transitioning from one parent to the other. In **oppositional defiant disorder**, the child is likely to be oppositional with both parents in a variety of contexts, while the child with **parental alienation disorder** is likely to focus his or her negativism on the proposed contact with the alienated parent and also to engage in the campaign of denigration of that parent.

When parents separate or divorce, a child may develop an **adjustment disorder** as a reaction to the various stressors related to the divorce including discord between the parents, the loss of a relationship with a parent, and the disruption of moving to a new neighborhood and school. A child with an **adjustment disorder** may have a variety of nonspecific symptoms including depression, anxious mood, and disruptive behaviors, while the child with **parental alienation disorder** manifests a specific cluster of symptoms including the campaign of denigration and weak, frivolous rationalizations for the child's persistent criticism of the alienated parent.

Parent-child relational problem (a V-code) is the appropriate diagnosis if the focus of clinical attention is on the relationship between a child and his or her divorced parents, but the symptoms do not meet the criteria for a mental disorder. For example, a rebellious adolescent may not have a specific mental disorder, but may temporarily refuse to have contact with one parent even though both parents have encouraged him to do so and a court has ordered it. On the other hand, **parental alienation disorder** should be the diagnosis if the child's symptoms are persistent enough and severe enough to meet the criteria for that disorder.

DIAGNOSTIC CRITERIA FOR
PARENTAL ALIENATION DISORDER

A. The child—usually one whose parents are engaged in a high-conflict divorce—allies himself or herself strongly with one parent and rejects a relationship with the other, alienated parent without legitimate justification. The child resists or refuses contact or parenting time with the alienated parent.

B. The child manifests the following behaviors:
   1. a persistent rejection or denigration of a parent that reaches the level of a campaign
   2. weak, frivolous, and absurd rationalizations for the child's persistent criticism of the rejected parent

C. The child manifests two or more of the following six attitudes and behaviors:
   1. lack of ambivalence
   2. independent-thinker phenomenon
   3. reflexive support of one parent against the other
   4. absence of guilt over exploitation of the rejected parent
   5. presence of borrowed scenarios
   6. spread of the animosity to the extended family of the rejected parent.

D. The duration of the disturbance is at least 2 months.

E. The disturbance causes clinically significant distress or impairment in social, academic (occupational), or other important areas of functioning.

F. The child's refusal to have contact with the rejected parent is without legitimate justification. That is, **parental alienation disorder** is not diagnosed if the rejected parent maltreated the child.

Appendix B

PROPOSED CRITERIA FOR PARENTAL ALIENATION RELATIONAL PROBLEM

This category should be used when the focus of clinical attention is a pattern of interaction between mother and child, father and child, and mother and father (e.g., the parents are divorced and the child forms a strong alliance with one parent [the preferred parent] and rejects a relationship with the other parent [the alienated parent] without legitimate justification) that is associated with clinically significant impairment in individual or family functioning or the development of clinically significant symptoms in parent or child.

The symptoms that typically occur in **parental alienation relational problem** are the child's persistent campaign of denigration against the alienated parent and weak, frivolous, and absurd rationalizations for the child's criticism of the alienated parent. The symptoms that sometimes occur in **parental alienation relational problem** include: lack of ambivalence (the child's belief that the alienated parent is all bad and the preferred parent is all good); the independent-thinker phenomenon (the child proudly states the decision to reject the alienated parent is his own, not influenced by the preferred parent); reflexive support of the preferred parent against the alienated parent; a disregard for the feelings of the alienated parent and an absence of guilt over exploitation of the alienated parent; borrowed scenarios (rehearsed statements that are identical to those made by the preferred parent); and the child's animosity toward the alienated parent may spread to that parent's extended family.

The diagnosis of **parental alienation relational problem** should not be used if the child's refusal to have contact with the rejected parent is justifiable, for example, if the child was neglected or abused by that parent.

Appendix C

LEGAL CITATIONS REGARDING
PARENTAL ALIENATION

The topics of parental alienation and PAS have been addressed in a large number of legal cases in the U.S., Canada, and other countries. Some of these cases are summarized in this appendix. This appendix is intended to be illustrative, not comprehensive. Also, the purpose of this appendix is not to show that the concepts of parental alienation and PAS have been accepted or rejected a certain number of times under *Frye* and *Daubert*. The purpose of this appendix is to show that courts frequently are required to deal with the problem of parental alienation, no matter what the phenomenon is called. Also, that courts are puzzled and hamstrung by the failure of the mental health community to develop standard definitions and criteria for the diagnosis of this common problem.

UNITED STATES

Alabama

Court of Civil Appeals

Ex parte S.C., 2009 Ala. Civ. App. LEXIS 449 (Ala. Civ. App. Aug. 14, 2009). After a divorce and custody settlement, the parents agreed to participate in counseling with the child. When visitation with the father became problematic, the child's counselor referred the child to a forensic psychologist who was an expert on PAS. The dispute in this proceeding involved issues with other counselors.

Goetsch v. Goetsch, 990 So. 2d 403 (Ala. Civ. App. 2008). After a divorce, the father had physical custody. The mother sought physical custody, alleging fear in the children and possible sexual abuse. The father introduced testimony of a psychologist who determined that the children suffered from PAS. The trial court placed little weight on the testimony because the psychologist had interviewed the children only once and obtained all her information from the father. The mother was awarded physical custody.

K.B. v. Cleburne County Department of Human Resources, 897 So. 2d 379 (Ala. Civ. App. 2004). An expert testified about PAS and said that it had not occurred in this case.

C.J.L. v. M.W.B., 879 So. 2d 1169 (Ala. Civ. App. 2003). If presented with the issue, the appellate court would be inclined to reject PAS under the *Frye* test for the admissibility of expert testimony about novel scientific theory. However, the appellate court found that the trial court used the concept of "parental alienation" when considering the parties' parental fitness and did not rely on a diagnosis of "parental alienation syndrome," which the court noted is not found in the *Diagnostic and Statistical Manual of Mental Disorders* (DMS-IV).

Alaska

Supreme Court

Pearson v. Pearson, 5 P.3d 239 (Alaska 2000). In this custody dispute, two experts testified about PAS, differing in their opinions as to whether it had occurred. The trial court made a factual finding that PAS had not occurred. On appeal, the father argued that the trial court erroneously disregarded his evidence and cited "a long list of cases from states and Canadian provinces sustaining decisions to admit evidence of the syndrome." The appellate court said the issue was irrelevant because the trial court allowed the expert testimony about PAS, even though "the theory is not universally accepted."

Court of Appeals

Plate v. Alaska, 925 P.2d 1057 (Alaska App. 1996). In a criminal case for sex crimes against the defendant's stepdaughter, the defendant asked for a psychological evaluation of the stepdaughter. In support of the request, an expert submitted an affidavit regarding PAS in blended families. The trial court ordered the evaluation, but at trial, the expert was only permitted to testify about the stepdaughter's factual statements, and not give an opinion about whether she was lying. The appellate court affirmed, because her veracity is a question of fact to be decided by the fact-finder.

Arkansas

Court of Appeals

Linder v. Johnson, 2006 Ark. App. LEXIS 780 (Ark. Ct. App. Nov. 29, 2006) (unpublished), *cert. denied,* 128 S. Ct. 69 (2007). After a divorce, the mother was awarded custody and the father was granted visitation. The father alleged that the mother systematically poisoned the children's minds against him. A psychologist found an "egregious" case of PAS and recommended a change of custody to the father. A different psychologist testified that PAS is not a "recognized diagnostic syndrome." The trial court changed custody to the father based on the mother's "egregious" conduct. The appellate court declined to address the acceptability of PAS as a diagnostic theory, holding that the trial court did not err in changing custody based on the facts.

Ignatiuk v. Ignatiuk, 2006 Ark. App. LEXIS 260 (Ark. Ct. App. April 12, 2006) (unpublished). In a custody dispute, the mother argued that recommendations of the children's guardian *ad litem* should be disregarded because of bias, unprofessionalism, and the fact that guardian *ad litem* changed her position on the theory of PAS. The experts did not address the issue of PAS. The appellate court said the trial court did not err in relying on the recommendations of the guardian *ad litem.*

Hanna v. Hanna, 2010 Ark App. LEXIS 72 (Ark. Ct. App. Jan. 20, 2010). The parents divorced after 20 years of marriage, and "the parties' two children were trapped in the no-man's land of the parties' internecine struggles." Both the trial court and the Court of Appeals discussed parental alienation–in the sense of the behavior of the alienating parent–as though the concept were fully accepted. The trial court found that the mother was "attempting parental alienation," so it changed the children's custody to the father. The Court of Appeals said the case involved parental alienation because "the custodial parent was apparently behind unfounded sexual-abuse allegations made against the noncustodial parent." The Court of Appeals affirmed the conclusions of the trial court.

California

Court of Appeals

In re John W., 41 Cal.App.4th 961, 48 Cal.Rptr.2d 899 (Cal. App. 1996). Allegations of abuse were made against father in juvenile court. Dr. Peter Chambers was appointed by the trial court to conduct an evaluation. The Court of Appeal stated, "Dr. Chambers concluded that *no* child abuse occurred. He blamed the mother for inducing the child to make statements indicating abuse. Chambers wrote, '[t]he allegations are a result of a subtle Parental Alienation Syndrome directed, at an unconscious level, by the minor's mother. . . .'" The issue of alienation was not addressed either by the trial court or by the review court. The matter was remanded to family court for determination of the best interests of the child as to custody.

Coursey v. Superior Court, 194 Cal.App.3d 147, 239 Cal.Rptr. 365 (Cal. App. 1987). In a divorce proceeding, the child's therapist, Katherine Moore, advised the court that the child suffered from "Parental Alienation Syndrome" and as a result did not wish to visit with her father. However, the court entered a visitation order and the child continued to refuse to visit father. The trial court found mother in contempt for the teenage daughter's refusal to visit. The Court of Appeal held that: (1) father failed to establish that mother had the ability to compel the 14-year-old daughter to visit with father as scheduled by the court order, and (2) father failed to establish that mother willfully violated the visitation order and, thus, mother could not be held in contempt. The issue of parental alienation was not addressed by the Court of Appeal.

Colorado

Court of Appeals

In re Marriage of Hatton, 160 P.3d 326 (Colo. Ct. App. March 8, 2007). After a divorce, the trial court ordered parenting time evaluations. The evaluator found that the children had become "enmeshed in mother's battle against father" and were not credible reporters because they were colluding with the mother to generate false allegations against the father. The evaluator recommended that the father be given all the parenting time and the mother be restricted from any contact. Although experts did not testify about PAS, the appellate court cited a study done in Colorado, which found that parental alienation occurred in 20 percent of cases involving custody disputes (quoting Kopetski, 1998a).

Connecticut

Court of Appeals

Ruggiero v. Ruggiero, 819 A.2d 864 (Conn. App. 2003). In this custody dispute, the appellate court distinguished between the trial court's factual finding of "parental alienation" versus a proposed mental health condition called "parental alienation syndrome," an "alleged psychiatric disorder" not listed in DSM-IV. Because the trial court made a factual finding, the appellate court declined to rule on the validity of PAS.

Superior Court

In re Jamie S., 2009 Conn. Super. LEXIS 754 (Conn. Super. Ct. March 9, 2009) (unpublished). The mother petitioned to terminate the father's parental rights, alleging abuse, abandonment, and refusal of the child to visit him. At the father's request, a psychologist examined the child and testified that "parental alienation" is a circumstance where one parent portrays the other parent in a negative light and the child takes note of such portrayal, and the child has no contact with the alienated parent based on the perception. Despite the testimony, the court terminated the father's parental rights because of mental health issues, substance abuse, emotional abuse, and abandonment.

Krukiel v. Krukiel, 2007 Conn. Super. LEXIS 166 (Conn. Super. Ct. Jan. 18, 2007) (unpublished). After a divorce, the mother had residential custody. The father sought residential custody, alleging that the mother alienated the children from him. The children's psychiatrist testified that there was a "state of alienation," exhibited by criteria such as unjustified antagonism and generalized negativity toward the alienated parent. The mother's expert criticized the psychiatrist's testimony, saying that it rested upon a diagnosis of PAS, "a syndrome yet to be recognized by the profession." The court said the psychiatrist's opinion was about a "state of alienation," not a diagnosis of "parental alienation syndrome." The father was awarded custody.

Synder v. Cedar, 2006 Conn. Super. LEXIS 520 (Conn. Super. Ct. Feb. 16, 2006) (unpublished). The father sued the mother for defamation, because of alleged statements to others that he was a child molester and for intentional infliction of emotional distress by causing the daughter to fabricate allegations of sexual contact. The father attempted to offer testimony of a psychologist that the child fabricated the allegations because of PAS. The court excluded testimony about PAS, finding that the theory had no scientific validity at this time.

Coleman v. Coleman, 2004 Conn. Super. LEXIS 2147 (Conn. Super. Ct. Aug. 5, 2004) (unpublished). In this custody dispute, the wife claimed that the husband was abusive and sexually assaulted her. The husband claimed that the wife used these allegations to alienate the children from him and obtain a tactical legal advantage in the custody case. The father argued that the children suffered from PAS, but offered no expert witness to establish its validity. The court said that Connecticut courts have not recognized PAS.

Metza v. Metza, 1998 Conn.Super LEXIS 2727 (Conn. Super. Ct. Sept. 25, 1998). In this custody dispute, a psychologist concluded in a report that the child had a risk of "parental alienation syndrome" from the mother's disparaging remarks about the father, and that the child exhibited "parental alienation." The court adopted the psychologist's conclusions as the court's conclusions, but awarded custody to the mother with an order not to make disparaging remarks in front of the child.

Bowles v. Bowles, 1997 Conn. Super. LEXIS 2721 (Conn. Super. Ct. Aug. 7, 1997) (unpublished). After their divorce, a mother and father had joint custody of the children. The older son wanted no contact with the father. Both parents filed motions to modify custody. There was lengthy testimony about PAS, whether it exists and, if so, whether it was present. The court declined to rule on the question because the court could determine custody based upon its own findings of fact, without regard to the theory.

Delaware

Family Court

D.M.W. v. T.V.W., 2005 Del. Fam. Ct. LEXIS 55 (Del. Fam. Ct. June 6, 2005). After a divorce, the mother had residential custody, and the father had visitation rights. The father sought shared residency, alleging that the mother was alienating the children from him. A psychologist performed a custody evaluation and found an "element of alienation." The mother hired another psychologist to review the evaluation, who testified that there is a "range of parental alienation syndrome." After hearing testimony from the experts, the court maintained primary residence with mother.

Ford v. Ford, 2000 Del. Fam. Ct. LEXIS 104 (Del. Fam. Ct. Dec. 19, 2000). Dr. Richard Gardner testified in this custody case. There were allegations of sexual abuse, but Dr. Gardner found no evidence of PAS.

Florida

Federal Court of Appeals

Marquard v. Secretary for Department of Corrections, 429 F.3d 1278 (11th Cir. 2005). During the sentencing phase of a murder case, the defendant introduced testimony of a forensic psychologist about the defendant's upbringing as a mitigating factor. The expert testified: "After talking to the mother and father, it became clear that there was a behavior pattern on both of their parts which we now refer to as Parental Alienation Syndrome. It's essentially when one parent, usually the custodial parent, does things or says things to the child or in front of the child which attempts, either consciously or unconsciously, to alienate the child from the other parent. At that time period, I don't believe there was terminology for that; but it's been a fairly common phenomenon for several years."

Hawaii

Intermediate Court of Appeals

Chee v. Chee, 2009 Haw. App. LEXIS 497 (Haw. Interm. Ct. App. June 19, 2009) (unpublished). After a divorce, the child resided with the father in Hawaii and the mother had visitation rights in Michigan. The child resisted returning to Hawaii after a visit. The mother and child alleged that the father sexually abused the child, which was determined to be unfounded. The father filed an *ex parte* motion for sole legal custody and submitted a letter from the child's psychologist stating that the child suffered from PAS. The trial court granted sole custody to the father without the mother's participation in the legal proceeding. The appellate court held that it was an error to proceed without the mother present.

Illinois

Supreme Court

In re Marriage of De Bates, 819 N.E.2d 714 (Ill. 2004). The trial court held a *Frye* hearing and ruled that PAS had gained general acceptance in the field of psychology, such that Dr. Richard Gardner and other experts could testify about it. However, the trial court said it would "throw out the words 'parental alienation syndrome'" and follow the language of the state statute governing the "best interest of child," in which a court must consider the "willingness and ability of each parent to facilitate and encourage a close and continuing relationship between the parents and child." On appeal, the Illinois Supreme Court declined to rule on the admissibility of the theory of PAS. Although the trial court ruled that the theory was admissible, the trial court did not rely on the theory of a "syndrome" in its ruling, so it was not an issue on appeal.

Indiana

Court of Appeals

In re Paternity of V.A.M.C., 768 N.E.2d 990 (Ind. App. 2002). In this custody dispute, the father thought the child was being sexually abused while in the mother's custody. An expert psychologist testified that the child should not go to the father because of a risk of "parental alienation" in the future. The father challenged the validity of the trial court's findings of fact, which were based on the expert's testimony, arguing that the expert relied on an inadmissible theory of "parental alienation syndrome." The appellate court rejected the argument, saying no diagnosis of PAS was made.

Kentucky

Federal District Court

Edwards v. Williams, 170 F. Supp. 2d 727 (E.D. Ky. 2001). In this case, government agency investigators were held not liable for violation of a parent's civil rights when they failed to investigate evidence of PAS after the daughter alleged abuse.

Louisiana

Court of Appeals

Palazzolo v. Mire, 10 So. 3d 748 (La. App. 2009). This was a custody and visitation dispute between a lesbian couple. The court did not rule on the validity of PAS as a scientific theory, but there is an extensive discussion of PAS, citing many legal and scientific sources.

White v. Kimrey, 847 So. 2d 157 (La. App. 2003). In this custody case, the mother made allegations of sexual abuse. The father's expert psychiatrist testified about PAS. The trial court accepted the expert's conclusions and awarded custody to the father. The issue of PAS was not challenged. On appeal, the appellate court modified the custody ruling to grant joint custody to the parents, with the father as the domiciliary parent.

Hollingsworth v. Semerad, 799 So. 2d 658 (La. App. 2001). In this visitation case, the father introduced expert testimony about PAS. Despite the testimony, the trial court found no evidence of parental alienation. The issue was not raised on appeal.

Maine

Federal District Court

Thun v. State, 2009 U.S. Dist. LEXIS 66670 (D. Maine July 28, 2009). This case involved federal review of a state conviction for sex crimes against a minor. The defendant argued ineffective assistance of his court-appointed lawyer, because the lawyer did not introduce testimony of an expert who would have testified that "there was a problem with the victim known as parental alienation syndrome." The state court held that, even if he had introduced the testimony, there is no indication that it would have been admitted because the defendant was not a parent of the victim. The federal judge agreed.

Maryland

Court of Special Appeals

Barton v. Hirschberg, 767 A.2d 874 (Md. Sp. App. 2001). In this custody dispute, a custody evaluator diagnosed the child with PAS, but recommended joint custody. The mother challenged the evaluator's reliance on the theory of PAS. The court said it would look at the facts, and the court did not rule on the theory of PAS.

Michigan

Federal District Court

Chee v. State, 2008 U.S. Dist. LEXIS 68004 (E.D. Mich. Sept. 8, 2008). The mother filed suit in Michigan federal court against various parties involved in child custody hearings in Hawaii, including a child psychologist, alleging denial of federal constitutional rights without due process of law. The psychologist had drafted a letter to the state court, saying the child suffered from PAS and should be with the father. The mother alleged this was "junk science" and she lost custody because of the psychologist's diagnosis. The federal court dismissed the claim for lack of jurisdiction.

Mississippi

Court of Appeals

Ellis v. Ellis, 952 So. 2d 982 (Miss. App. 2006). After a divorce, the mother had physical custody. The father sought custody, alleging that the mother had interfered with his visitation rights and alienated the child from him. One psychologist testified that the child was alienated from the father, but the alienation was caused by the father's own behavior. Another psychologist testified that the child suffered from PAS, "a systematic programmed alienation of a child from one parent brought upon by the other parent," and that the alienation was caused by the mother. The second psychologist recommended a change of custody to the father. The court looked at factors governing the "best interest of the child" as required by statute and changed custody to the father.

Nevada

Supreme Court

Truax v. Truax, 874 P.2d 10 (Nev. 1994). The Nevada supreme court noted, "The litigants have been fighting over the custody of their three children for the pat several years. This fight has been the stage for a myriad of allegations, formal charges, and official court battles." The father's expert, Dr. Elizabeth Richitt, testified that the children were victims of "coaching" and "parental alienation syndrome." Another expert, Dr. Lewis Etcoff, concluded there was no evidence of parental alienation syndrome. The supreme court affirmed the order of the district court, which gave primary physical custody to the mother and visitation rights to the father.

New Jersey

Superior Court

Coles v. Pinn-Wilson, 2008 N.J. Super. Unpub. LEXIS 1452 (N.J. Super. Ct. March 26, 2008) (unpublished). The mother sought to modify a custody decree from joint custody to sole custody. The father filed a cross-motion to enforce his parenting time, alleging that the mother's malicious interference with his exercise of parenting rights had resulted in PAS. The court found that the rupture in the relationship between the father and child was mostly due to the father's own actions.

New York

Federal District Court

Daniels v. Murphy, 2007 U.S. Dist. LEXIS 47838 (E.D.N.Y. July 2, 2007). The mother filed a suit in federal court against various parties involved in a state court custody matter, alleging denial of federal constitutional rights without due process of law. The mother claimed that the father intimidated the child, engaged in "brainwashing and Parental Alienation Syndrome," and made fraudulent statements to child protective services. The federal court dismissed the suit for failure to state a federal claim.

Supreme Court, Appellate Division

Smith v. Bombard, 741 N.Y.S.2d 336 (N.Y. Sup. Ct. App. Div. 2002). In this custody dispute, the father sought sole custody of the daughters, alleging that the mother was alienating them from him. The mother had two expert psychologists testify that the daughters' refusal to see their father was not the result of PAS. The court retained custody with the mother.

In the matter of Krebsbach v. Gallagher, 587 N.Y.S.2d 346 (N.Y. Sup. Ct. App. Div. 1992). An expert psychiatrist testified that there was no evidence of PAS. The testimony was not challenged.

Supreme Court, Kings County

N.K. v. M.K., 851 N.Y.S.2d 71 (N.Y. Sup. Ct., Kings County Oct. 1, 2007) (unpublished). After a divorce, the mother had custody and the father had visitation rights, but the child refused to visit him. This case involved distribution of the marital assets and the father asked the court to take into account the child's refusal to visit him, which he alleged was due to the mother's pattern of alienation. The court declined to grant the father economic relief because of the child's refusal to visit. The court did not believe there is a generally accepted diagnostic syndrome known as "parental alienation syndrome," saying that a term such as "inappropriate parental influence" would be more appropriate (citing Hoult, 2006).

Miscellaneous

People v. Bimonte, 712 N.Y.S.2d 829 (N.Y. City Crim. Ct. 2000). Expert testimony about PAS was not allowed in this sex crime case. The court held that such testimony is only relevant in a custody dispute.

People v. Loomis, 658 N.Y.S.2d 787 (N.Y. County Ct., Suffolk County 1997). Testimony regarding PAS was held inadmissible in this criminal case.

North Dakota

Supreme Court

In the Interest of T.T., 681 N.W.2d 779 (N.D. June 30, 2004). In an action by the state human services department to place a child in state custody, the state's expert witness testified about PAS, opining that both parents were guilty of alienating behaviors and the mother was an "obsessed alienator." The mother objected, arguing that the expert did not have enough experience to testify about PAS. The trial court allowed the testimony. On appeal, the mother argued that PAS is not a recognized scientific disorder. The appellate court did not allow the mother to assert that position on appeal because she failed to raise it during the trial.

Ohio

Court of Appeals

Weisgarber v. Weisgarber, 2009 Ohio App. LEXIS 4 (Ohio Ct. App. Jan. 5, 2009). In this case, the mother sought to terminate the father's visitation rights, alleging that visitation frightened the children and the father exposed the children to abuse from an uncle. The father sought custody, alleging that the mother alienated the children. A psychologist's report said "seven of eight identifying factors of PAS or parental alienation syndrome" were present. The court relied on the report, along with other evidence, to find that the mother had engaged in a pattern of parental alienation. The court granted custody to the father.

In the matter of J.M., 2008 Ohio App. LEXIS 5631 (Ohio Ct. App. Dec. 22, 2008). During a divorce and custody battle, the father alleged that the children suffered from PAS caused by the mother turning the children against him. The court agreed that therapy with a psychologist was necessary to identify the existence of PAS and whether the children needed specific treatment before they could be reunited with the father. This case deals with payment of the psychologist's bills.

Truex v. Truex, 901 N.E.2d 259 (Ohio App. 2008). A psychologist conducted a psychological evaluation for PAS. The mother asked for a continuance of the case, saying she did not have sufficient time to review the psychological report. The court denied the continuance because the delay was due to the mother's own failure to cooperate with the psychological evaluation.

Cichanowicz v. Cichanowicz, 2008 Ohio App. LEXIS 4023 (Ohio Ct. App. Sept. 22, 2008). After a divorce, the mother had residential custody and the father sought residential custody. A custody evaluator was appointed, who found evidence of PAS and recommended a change of custody to the father. The court found the report unacceptable because the evaluator relied on information supplied by the father without interviewing the mother. The court said, even if PAS existed in this case, the case did not exhibit the type of egregious conduct that had warranted a change in custody as found in other cases in which psychologists testified about parental alienation.

Hamilton v. Hamilton, 2008 Ohio App. LEXIS 3138 (Ohio Ct. App. July 25, 2008). In this custody dispute, the father's expert psychologist testified that the children suffered from PAS, but based this conclusion only on the father's information without interviewing the children or the mother. The court found the testimony of other witnesses more credible, who testified that the mother was more fit as a parent.

Horning v. Wolff, 2006 Ohio App. LEXIS 6345 (Ohio Ct. App. Dec. 4, 2006). In this custody dispute, a psychologist conducted a "parental alienation evaluation" for the court. The psychologist found that the child exhibited PAS and the mother would not facilitate any relationship between the child and the father, absent court intervention. The court awarded custody to the father.

Curie v. Curie, 2006 Ohio App. LEXIS 6058 (Ohio Ct. App. Nov. 17, 2006). In this custody dispute, a psychologist testified that there was strong evidence of PAS. The mother was ignoring court orders granting the father visitation, so the court placed the children in state custody pending a forensic evaluation for parental alienation. Another psychologist conducted the forensic evaluation and found that "this case meets every criteria of Parental Alienation Syndrome" and recommended that the father have custody. The issue on appeal involved procedural matters regarding legal representation of the children.

In the Matter of S.G., 2003 Ohio App. LEXIS 109 (Ohio Ct. App. Jan. 16, 2003). In this custody dispute, a psychologist testified that the mother's family exhibited a "campaign of denigration" of the father, indicating the existence of PAS. Despite this testimony, the trial court awarded custody to the mother. The testimony about PAS was not challenged. The appellate court reversed the decision for abuse of discretion and remanded the case back to the trial court for a determination of the child's best interest.

Doerman v. Doerman, 2002 Ohio App. LEXIS 3183 (Ohio Ct. App. June 24, 2002). In this custody dispute, a psychologist testified about PAS, including differentiating between "moderate" and "severe" PAS. The mother made unsubstantiated allegations of abuse by the father, thwarted visitation, coached the children's conversations on the phone, and disregarded court orders. The court found evidence of severe PAS and awarded custody to the father.

In re Adoption of Wagner, 1999 Ohio App. LEXIS 3117 (Ohio Ct. App. June 30, 1999). In this adoption case, the biological father, who appeared *pro se,* opposed adoption of the child. The father's new wife, who had some psychology training, testified that the children did not see their biological father due to PAS. The trial court limited the father's ability to introduce evidence. The appellate court reversed and remanded for a new proceeding, stating that the father should be allowed to present evidence, but any testimony about PAS would need to be admissible under the rules of evidence.

Arthur v. Arthur, 720 N.E.2d 176 (Ohio App. 1998). In this custody dispute, a court-appointed psychologist testified that he recommended shared parenting to avoid the development of PAS, due to a lack of cooperation between the husband and wife. The testimony about PAS was not challenged.

Pisani v. Pisani, 1998 Ohio App. LEXIS 4421 (Ohio Ct. App. Sept. 24,

1998). In this visitation dispute, a psychologist filed a report with the court. Later, the court denied a request to hold a hearing where the psychologist could testify regarding PAS. The appellate court affirmed, stating that the trial court has broad discretion in visitation matters and already considered the psychologist's report.

Conner v. Renz, 1995 Ohio App. LEXIS 176 (Ohio Ct. App. Jan. 19, 1995). In this custody dispute, an expert psychologist provided a report detailing evidence of PAS, and a hearing was held on the issue. The hearing was objected to on due process grounds because of a lack of notice of the PAS claim prior to the hearing. The court rejected the due process argument.

Sims v. Hornsby, 1992 Ohio App. LEXIS 4074 (Ohio Ct. App. Aug. 10, 1992). In this case, an expert provided testimony at trial about PAS. There was no objection to the testimony.

Oklahoma

Supreme Court

Kaiser v. Kaiser, 23 P.3d 278 (Okla. 2001). In this case, the mother requested to modify the visitation schedule so that she could move out of the state. The father opposed, and he introduced testimony of a psychologist about PAS in general, but the psychologist had not interviewed the parties. The testimony was not challenged. The court did not rely on the testimony, and it granted the mother's motion.

Pennsylvania

Federal District Court

Dreibelbis v. Young, 2007 U.S. Dist. LEXIS 90659 (M.D. Pa. Dec. 10, 2009). The father filed suit in federal court against various parties involved in state custody hearings. He alleged denial of federal constitutional rights without due process of law because he was not permitted to videotape a visit with the child, which was supervised by a court-appointed child services agency. The father claimed he needed to videotape the encounter so that it could be evaluated by an expert capable of diagnosing PAS. The federal court declined to exercise jurisdiction because the issues had already been litigated in state court.

Texas

Court of Appeals

Rangel v. State, 2007 Tex. App. LEXIS 4761 (Tex. Ct. App. June 17, 2007) (unpublished), *review denied, In re Rangel,* 2008 Tex. Crim. App. LEXIS 135 (Tex. Crim. App. Jan. 23, 2008). In this criminal case for sexual abuse of a minor by her uncle, the defendant attempted to introduce a defense of PAS. On cross-examination, the state's expert psychologist testified that he was familiar with the term "parental alienation syndrome" and that "it has to do with a way that children can be inappropriately pressured to make false allegations of child sexual abuse." The court held that the defense did not apply to this case, because the defendant was not the victim's parent, and because the theory is generally raised in family law cases.

Virginia

Federal District Court

Shaw v. Lynchburg Dept. of Soc. Services, 2009 U.S. Dist. LEXIS 6659 (W.D. Va. Jan. 29, 2009). The mother sued various lawyers, social workers, and psychologists in federal court, alleging denial of her federal due process rights during state custody hearings. She alleged that the parties suppressed evidence of sexual abuse and created a false perception that the children were suffering from PAS. The court noted: "The parental alienation syndrome is a disorder that arises primarily in the context of child-custody disputes. Its primary manifestation is the child's campaign of denigration against a parent, a campaign that has no justification. It results from the combination of a programming (brainwashing) parent's indoctrinations and the child's own contributions to the vilification of the target parent" (quoting Gardner, 1998b). The federal court declined to exercise jurisdiction because the issues were already considered in the custody hearings.

Court of Appeals

Ange v. Chesapeake Dep't of Human Services, 1998 Va. App. LEXIS 59 (Va. Ct. App. Feb. 3, 1998). In this case, the department of human services petitioned the court to terminate the biological father's parental rights to a child in foster care. The father asked that custody with an aunt be considered. A psychologist testified that the child suffered from PAS due to the aunt's interference with the child's relationship with the foster parents. There was no challenge to the testimony about PAS. The court terminated the father's parental rights.

Wisconsin

Court of Appeals

Fischer v. Fischer, 584 N.W.2d 233 (Wis. App. 1998). In this custody dispute, experts testified that the mother was engaged in conduct to undermine the relationship of the child with his father, and that the son should be placed with the father if the mother's behavior escalates to the level of PAS. There was no challenge to the testimony of PAS. The trial court awarded custody to the father. The appellate court affirmed.

Janell S. v. J.R.S., 571 N.W.2d 924 (Wis. App. 1997). In this custody dispute, the mother alleged that the father was physically abusing the child. The father's expert psychologist testified that the child exhibited PAS. For procedural reasons related to the court's schedule, the court did not allow testimony of a social worker to rebut the testimony of PAS. The appellate court reversed, allowing the social worker to testify that the child did not suffer from PAS.

Wyoming

Supreme Court

Carlton v. Carlton, 997 P.2d 1028 (Wyo. 2000). In this divorce and custody case, the son did not want to live with the father. The father presented expert testimony that the son suffered from PAS. A counselor who treated the son testified that PAS does not exist, and recommended that the mother be awarded custody. The court accepted the testimony of the counselor and awarded custody to the mother.

McCoy v. State, 886 P.2d 252 (Wyo. 1994). In a criminal case, the defense counsel was not ineffective in failing to introduce expert testimony of PAS as a defense.

CANADA

Alberta

Court of Appeal

Elliott v. Elliott, A.J. No. 1065 (Alberta Ct. App., Nov. 7, 1996). In this custody dispute, the father had residential custody. The mother's expert psychologist testified that the child was at risk for PAS because of the father's disparaging attitudes. The trial judge explained that the central issue in dispute was the effect of PAS. The trial judge wanted to prevent impairment of the child's relationship with the mother in the future because custody law requires courts to promote a relationship with both parents. The trial judge switched residential custody to the mother. The decision was affirmed on appeal.

Court of Queen's Bench

R.A.L. v. R.D.R., A.J. No. 163 (Alberta Ct. Queen's Bench, Feb. 7, 2007). In this custody dispute, the mother sought sole custody, alleging that the father alienated the child. The father's expert testified that "parental alienation" exists only when certain criteria are met, such as unqualified hatred of the "bad" parent, and the child's words are not his or her own. The court rejected this definition and accepted the testimony of the mother's expert, who said "parental alienation" occurs along a continuum of behaviors, and it is not necessary to find a certain number of criteria.

F.D.R. v. M.D.P., A.J. No. 1502 (Alberta Ct. Queen's Bench, Dec. 20, 2004). In this custody dispute, the father had interim residential custody. The mother sought residential custody. The father alleged that the mother suffered from mental illness and had sexually abused the child. The mother argued that the child suffered from PAS. The court explained: "Parental alienation syndrome describes a situation in which one parent attempts to alienate the child against the other parent." The court accepted the testimony of an expert psychologist about parental alienation and the expert's recommendation that the mother be awarded custody.

New Brunswick

Court of Queen's Bench

Jefferson v. Jefferson, N.B.J. No. 11 (New Brunswick Ct. Queen's Bench, Jan. 18, 2000). In this custody dispute, the father sought custody of the child. The mother argued that the child suffered from PAS and offered expert psychological testimony. The court stated: "Although much was said about parental alienation syndrome, there is nothing conclusive, and if it is present in this case, it is at a worrisome but not extreme stage." The court denied the father's petition for custody, and the child remained with the mother.

S.O. v. S.C.O., N.B.J. No. 326 (New Brunswick Ct. Queen's Bench, July 30, 1999). In this custody dispute, the father had custody of the children. The mother petitioned for custody. A psychologist testified that the children suffered from PAS. The psychologist differentiated between "moderate" and "severe" PAS and how the designation affects custody. The court found evidence of severe alienation and awarded custody to the mother.

Newfoundland

Unified Family Court

Toope v. Toope, N.J. No. 182 (Newfoundland Unified Fam. Ct., June 15, 2000). In this custody dispute, the mother sought to introduce recordings of phone conversations between the father and child that she illegally recorded, as evidence of PAS. The court allowed the recordings into evidence to shed light on the parental alienation issue, even though they were obtained illegally.

Nova Scotia

Family Court

Badakhshan v. Moradi, N.S.J. No. 605 (Nova Scotia Fam. Ct., Mar. 2, 1993). In this custody dispute, the court noted that there was no evidence to suggest that the children were suffering from PAS. The court distinguished this case from the case of *Mills v. Cher,* No. 500-12-184613-895 (Quebec Super. Ct. Feb. 15, 1991), in which the father strongly influenced the children against their mother, and the children had become severely alienated from their mother, to the point of totally rejecting her. In the *Mills* case, a psychological opinion was introduced that the children were suffering from PAS.

Ontario

Superior Court of Justice

Pettenuzzo-Deschene v. Deschene, O.J. No. 3062 (Ontario Super. Ct. Just., Aug. 10, 2007). In this case, the mother had custody of the children. The father sought custody, alleging that the mother persistently denied his access. A psychologist testified that the children suffered from PAS. The court quoted Dr. Richard Gardner's definition of PAS as "the definition generally accepted in the psychology community." The court awarded temporary custody to the father, wanting time for the father and children to re-establish relationships without the mother's influence.

C.S. v. M.S., O.J. No. 787 (Ontario Super. Ct. Just., Feb. 27, 2007). In this case, the mother sought a court order restraining the father from contacting the child, who was in the mother's custody, because of a pattern of parental alienation. The mother offered an article on PAS into evidence, but her expert psychologist did not explain the theory. The judge decided not to attach a formal label of "syndrome" to the situation, but he considered the concept in making findings of fact. The judge issued a restraining order against the father prohibiting his access to the child.

R. v. K.C., O.J. No. 3162 (Ontario Super. Ct. Just., Aug. 9, 2002). In this criminal case against a father for charges of sexual abuse of his daughters, Dr. Richard Gardner testified about PAS. The mother and father had been involved in a contentious divorce. The court found Dr. Gardner's testimony relevant and admissible, but the court "did not have to rely on it" in rendering its decision. The defendant was found not guilty because the children were not credible witnesses. The judge attached a full article by Dr. Gardner about PAS as an exhibit to the opinion: "I attach this because it does appear that the subject of Dr. Gardner's theories are beginning to occur in our courts . . . and I suspect we in the court system may be hearing more about it in the future, particularly in child custody proceedings."

Orszak v. Orszak, O.J. No. 1606 (Ontario Super. Ct. Just., May 5, 2000). In this custody dispute, the court ordered that visitation time with the father be gradually increased, to "overcome what may be parental alienation syndrome which has been developing over the past while."

Fortin v. Major, O.J. No. 3805 (Ontario Ct. Just., Oct. 25, 1996). In this case, the father sought a court order forcing the child to visit him and forcing her to seek counseling with a therapist who specialized in PAS. Dr. Richard Gardner testified that the child suffered from PAS. An opposing expert disagreed. The court accepted the testimony of the opposing expert and held that it would not be in child's best interest to force visitation or counseling.

Davy v. Davy, O.J. No. 2451 (Ontario Ct. Just., Oct. 7, 1993). In this case, the father petitioned for increased visitation. The children said they hated their father and did not want to see him. An expert psychologist testified that the children suffered from PAS and that the children had been programmed by their mother to hate the father. The court granted the father increased visitation access.

Quebec

Superior Court

R.F. v. S.P. [2000] Q.J. No. 3412 (Quebec Super. Ct., Oct. 13, 2000). In this custody dispute, a father sought sole custody. An expert social worker testified that the child suffered from PAS. The expert cited the work of Dr. Richard Gardner and described the criteria of PAS. The father, sister, and brother all cited verbatim a list of grievances against the mother, and the mother was seen as "all bad," while the father was seen as "all good." The court denied the father's request for sole custody but ordered that the parents stop denigrating each other.

Mills v. Cher, No. 500-12-184613-895 (Quebec Super. Ct., Feb. 15, 1991) (unpublished). This case is mentioned in *Badakhshan v. Moradi,* N.S.J. No. 605 (Nova Scotia Fam. Ct., Mar. 2, 1993). In *Mills,* the father strongly influenced the children against their mother, and the children had become severely alienated from their mother, to the point of totally rejecting her. A psychological opinion was introduced that the children were suffering from PAS. Judge John H. Gomery said, "Hatred is not an emotion that comes naturally to a child. It has to be taught. The person who has taught the children [in this case] is their father. They would be better off if he were to be removed as an influence upon their development until they are better able to withstand and reject his negative attitudes. . . . Defendant has deliberately poisoned the minds of his children against the mother that they formerly loved and needed. In the Court's opinion, a father who would act in this way represents a grave and persistent danger to the mental and emotional health of his children."

EUROPEAN COURT OF HUMAN RIGHTS

Bianci v. Switzerland, No. 7548/04 (European Ct. Human Rights, Sept. 22, 2006). A bi-national couple (Italian father, Swiss mother) lived in Italy. After they separated, the mother abducted their 3-year-old boy from Italy to Switzerland. The Italian court gave custody of the child to the father. Also, the federal Court of Switzerland ordered the return of the child to Italy. However, one year later, the mother abducted the child a second time. The father sued in the European Court of Human Rights (ECtHR), and that court agreed that the Swiss authorities failed to take adequate measures to bring about the return of the child to Italy and to the custodial father. The court decided that the father's family law rights under the European Convention on Human Rights were violated. The ECtHR said: "This passivity [of the Swiss authorities] is the origin of the total rupture of the relation between father and child, which lasted nearly two years and which implicates–in this child of a very young age–the risk of increasing alienation between the two, alienation that cannot be considered at all consistent with the best interest of the child."

C. v. Finland, No. 18249/02 (European Ct. Human Rights, May 9, 2006). After a divorce, the mother had custody of the children along with the mother's female partner. When the mother died, her female partner retained custody. The father sought custody, alleging that the female partner manipulated the children to turn against him. The trial court awarded custody to the father, but the children refused to see him. An appellate court also awarded custody to the father. The Supreme Court of Finland, however, awarded custody to the female partner, finding that the children's desire to stay with her was their own independent wish. The father sued in the European Court of Human Rights at Strasbourg, which held that the Supreme Court's action violated the father's family law rights under the European Convention on Human Rights. The legal issue was that the manipulated child's expressed desire should not be accepted as his or her real desire, that is, the manipulated child is not competent to give informed consent.

Koudelka v. Czech Republic, No. 1633/05 (European Ct. Human Rights, July 20, 2006). After a divorce, the mother had custody of the child in the Czech Republic. The father sued in Czech courts to enforce his visitation rights, alleging that the mother prevented him from seeing the child. Experts testified that the mother had been "instilling a parental alienation syndrome in the child" and noted a "pathological fixation on the mother." The Czech courts issued warnings to the mother to allow visitation, but the father alleged that the Czech courts failed to enforce his rights. He sued in the European Court on Human Rights at Strasbourg, which agreed that the Czech courts failed to enforce the father's family law rights as required by the European Convention on Human Rights.

Kutzner v. Germany, No. 46544/99 (European Ct. Human Rights, February 26, 2002). Two children were taken from their parents into compulsory public custody on the grounds of mental retardation of the parents, with minimal contact between the parents and the children and between the children themselves. No physical or emotional abuse had been found, but the authorities were afraid that the parents could not properly take care of the children in the long run. Although the German courts approved the public custody, the European Court of Human Rights did not. In its decision, the Court alluded to parental alienation: "Having regard to the fact that the children were very young, severing contact in this way and imposing such restrictions on visiting rights could, in the Court's opinion, only lead to the children's increased alienation [Entfremdung] from the parents and from each other." This is an example of parental alienation induced by authorities such as social service workers.

Zavrel v. Czech Republic, No. 14044/05 (European Ct. Human Rights, Jan. 18, 2007). After a divorce, the mother had custody. The father sued in the Czech court system, alleging that the mother prevented him from exercising his visitation rights. Experts testified that the child exhibited "early signs of parental alienation syndrome." The experts recommended expanding the father's visitation rights. Czech courts sent formal warnings to the mother, but the father alleged the Czech courts failed to enforce his rights, so he sued in the European Court of Human Rights at Strasbourg, which agreed that the Czech courts failed to enforce the father's family law rights as required by the European Convention on Human Rights.

FRANCE

M. v. G., Case No. 04/00694, Tribunal de Grande Instance de Toulon (JAF), June 4, 2007. This case from an appellate court was published in *La Gazette du Palais* 127 (322–324) 11–15, November 18–20, 2007. Based on testimony by a psychological expert, it was decided that the two children were victims of Parental Alienation Syndrome, induced by their mother. The children had severe psychological consequences, which were described in detail. The court accorded visitation rights ("droit de visite et d'hébergement progressif") to the father, so that their relationship could be reconstructed. The court said, "Il est urgent de faire cesser cette dictature affective qui pèse sur les enfants." ("It is urgent to stop this emotional dictatorship which is a burden for the children.")

GERMANY

Anonymous v. Anonymous, Case No. 2 XV 178, Amtsgericht Rinteln, April 27, 1998. This case from a circuit court was published in *Zentralblatt für Jugendrecht* 85 (7/8) 344–346, 1998. This was the first family court decision regarding PAS in Germany, which discussed "parental alienation syndrome" in detail. The "parental alienation syndrome in its classical form" was diagnosed by the psychological expert. The court gave visitation to the father of a 9-year-old boy against the wishes of the mother and against the declared opinion of the child. The court decided that it was not in the best interests of the child to follow the mother's wish for no contact between father and son, and that the child was obviously severely manipulated by his mother against the father.

Sch. v. Sch., Case No. 17 UF 1413/99, Kammergericht Berlin, May 30, 2000. This case from an appellate court was published in FamRZ 47 (24) 1606-07, 2000. The court decided to give custody of a 10-year-old child and a 12-year-old child to the mother, against the will of the father and against the will of the two children. An expert in child psychiatry testified regarding parental alienation syndrome, which was caused by the father's programming and influencing the children.

Anonymous v. Anonymous, Case No. 6 WF 168/00, Oberlandesgericht Frankfurt am Main, October 26, 2000. This case from an appellate court was published on *www.hefam.de/urteile/6WF16800.html.* The mother of 10-year-old and 12-year-old girls refused to allow the father to have any contact with daughters without adequate reason. The girls did not want to see their father. The mother also refused to cooperate in the court-ordered psychological evaluation and in mediation. The court decided that the mother was abusing her role as custodial parent and that she did psychological harm to the children. Parental alienation syndrome was mentioned by the court, which threatened a change of custody if the mother did not change her attitude and her contact-refusing behavior.

Anonymous v. Anonymous, Case No. 6 UF 4/05, Oberlandesgericht Zweibrücken, May 9, 2005. This case from an appellate court was published in *FamRZ* 53 (2) 144–145, 2006. The court heard detailed testimony from a psychological expert. The mother had refused to allow the children, age 8 and 9, to have contact with their father over six years. The court decided that the mother had severely influenced the children to have unrealistic and distorted negative beliefs, which had been consciously inculcated by her. The court said that the severe alienation process had led to a psychological disorder in both children in the sense of parental alienation syndrome. The court recommended psychological consultation to the mother and appointed a guardian *ad litem* to help the children to reconstruct their relationship with their father.

ITALY

A case (No. 1652/E/97) at the Juvenile Court in Milan (June 19, 1998), which was the first legal case in Italy regarding PAS. A minor, who declared his wish to continue living with his father, was assigned to social services based of the advice of an expert witness. According to the Court, it seriously injured the child to be in the father's custody. The Court said, ". . . the relationship established between father and son was seriously detrimental to the psychological integrity of the child. Indeed, the child's attitude was becoming increasingly paranoid, as that of the father. The child appeared to suffer from what some experts call parental alienation syndrome. . . ."

A case before the Judge for Preliminary Investigations of Treviso (October 12, 2007). The court indicted a mother "for the crime under article 572 of the Criminal Code [Abuse in the Family or to Children] for mistreating her children and maintaining toward them patterns of systematic denigration and contempt for the father, which made the children feel extreme discomfort and emotional distress and caused a serious form of parental alienation, with pathological manifestations typical of a severe degree of PAS (Parental Alienation Syndrome)."

SPAIN

Anonymous v. Anonymous, Case No. 567/06, Sentencia del Juzgado de Primera Instancia número 4 de Manresa, June 14, 2007. This case from a trial court was published on *www.separaciones-divorcios.com/noticias/index.php?id =31.* The mother had hateful feelings toward the father and programmed their 8-year-old daughter against him. The court changed custody and gave it to the father. For the next six months, mother and her extended family were not allowed to have contact with the girl. Until the change of residence could be accomplished, the child lived with the paternal grandparents as a transition.

SWEDEN

Linköpings tingsrätt, Case No. T 3695-06, May 21, 2007. In this case, the trial court stated: "[Mother] has had obvious difficulties in telling why [Father] is not suitable to take care of the children. Above all, it seems to consist of his wanting to take away her control over the children. [Father] is surely sincere in his conviction that it is a case of PAS and that radical actions have to be taken to solve this. . . . Today the children seem to have a very negative picture of [Father]. That there is any factual foundation for this has not been demonstrated in the case. The court can today see no other possibility for the reconnection between the children and [Father] other than giving sole custody to [Father]. The court presupposes thereby that [Mother], after a transition period when the relation between the father and the children are established, will be given reasonable visitation rights." This verdict was overturned by an appellate court.

Göteborgs tingsrätt, Case No. T 3406-06, July 13, 2007. In this case, the trial court stated: "It has been made clear that [Child] during all the years when he was growing up has been imprinted by the conflict between his parents. He has thereby been influenced by his mother to have a negative attitude toward his father. The mother has with all available means tied [Child] to herself in a way that stands out as damaging." The court gave sole custody to the child's father.

Södertälje tingsrätt, Case No. T 2562-07, March 20, 2009. In this case, the trial court stated: "The different reported accusations [Mother] has made have not ended up in any other result than the children have had to live a turbulent life with recurrent investigations and obscure living conditions. The court cannot come to any other conclusion than the one that [Mother's] suspicions and attitude toward [Father] entails that the children are badly treated and that the children are not allowed to have a natural contact with their father. . . . Taken into consideration the infected situation for the parties and considering the accusations put forward, the Court finds it important to give custody to that parent who can best see to the children's need to have a natural and extensive contact with the other parent. Thereby the children can feel allied to both parents, something that is important for the children's development. The investigation in the case gives strong support for the conclusion that [Father] is the parent who can see that the children will have continuous contact with the other parent." The trial court gave sole custody to the father.

Solna tingsrätt, Case No. T 8421-07, April 24, 2009. In this case, the trial court stated: "The court notes that these words, 'not force a child,' is an odd expression often coming up in custody cases. Custody is about guiding, taking care of, and deciding for children. To choose the word, 'force,' is to put something negative into what is a custodian's self-evident responsibility. . . . The responsibility for how the children behave does not end with the adult's reference to the child's will. If the child's will were superior to all other considerations, then the child doesn't need a custodian. . . . The children–by being moved from their home, by being prevented from having a normal contact with their father, by not having any undisturbed space with him, by being subjected to their mother's denigration of their father–have been at the mercy of their mother and her picture of their father. . . . The psychologist, Lena Hellblom Sjögren, has in her investigation and in her testimony in a systematic and knowledgeable manner demonstrated how the children's situation gradually has developed in an unhealthy manner and that it is governed by the mother's hostility. Even if the process is not given a summarized name as PAS, Parental Alienation Syndrome, the way of acting is not new in history or from the viewpoint of the Court's experience. Men and women, fathers and mothers, who unconsciously or more or less deliberately act to shut out and denigrate the other as a parent as a person and who use the children as tools is something that happens now and then." The trial court gave sole custody to the father. The verdict was overturned by an appellate court, and the case will be tried again.

SWITZERLAND

Anonymous v. Anonymous, Case no. 220126, *Obergericht des Kantons Luzern,* March 6, 2002. This case was heard by an appellate court. The court noted a high degree of conflict between the parents in nearly all aspects of daily life of the three children, a 13-year-old boy, an 11-year-old girl, and a 9-year-old boy. An expert in child psychiatry had diagnosed parental alienation syndrome, which had been induced by the father. The court took custody away from both parents and transferred it to a social worker, who also functioned as a supervisor for the parents. The children's residence remained provisionally with the father and extended visitation rights were ordered for the mother. The court wanted to observe if its custody decision, the supervising support by the social worker, and the visitation ordered for the mother would bring about improved cooperation by the parents and normalize the relationships of the children with their mother.

UNITED KINGDOM

Re: C (Prohibition of Further Applications), 1 FLR 1136, 3 FCR 183 (Ct. App. Civ. Div., Feb. 20 , 2002). In this case, the father sought joint custody, but the child refused to see him. The father petitioned the court to appoint a psychologist who was an expert on PAS to evaluate the child. The petition was denied, as was joint custody. On appeal, the appellate court believed the father's view of PAS obscured other more obvious reasons why the child refused to visit him. The court ordered an evaluation of the family by a mental health expert "to see whether there is any way out of their problems and not to concentrate upon the issue of parental alienation syndrome."

V v. V, In the High Court of Justice, Family Division (May 20, 2004). This custody and visitation dispute had been addressed in several courts over several years, in that the father repeatedly claimed that the mother interfered with his relationship with their two children. Mrs. Justice Bracewell wrote an eloquent overview of how the courts deal with this type of intractable problem. She then summarized the chronology of this case. Although she did not use the words "parental alienation," that is what she described in detail. In her conclusions, Mrs. Justice Bracewell said, "I make findings of fact as follows: that each of the allegations made by the mother against the father and his family are either false or wholly exaggerated out of all proportion. I find the mother has made allegations to frustrate contact and in order to do so has coached the children, involved them in false allegations, and has subjected them to emotional abuse. . . . That abuse is likely to continue while she has the care of the children. . . . Having considered all the factors, weighing all the risks and advantages, I am satisfied that the need for these children to have a relationship with their father can only be met by transferring residence to him."

Appendix D

PARENTAL ALIENATION
AND THE GENERAL PUBLIC

The general public is the intended audience for the following publications, media products, and websites. Nonprofessionals have created and contributed to these print, broadcast, and online resources in an effort to educate others and help parents and children avoid the pain and heartache that they have experienced due to parental alienation. This section does not include the thousands of individual newspaper articles, magazine articles, and Internet articles regarding parental alienation and PAS. A Google search of the phrase "parental alienation" produced 168,000 hits. A search for "parental alienation" by LexisNexis in "Major U.S. and World Publications" (which primarily taps large newspapers) produced more than 300 articles.

BOOKS

The following books, intended for the general public, were written by nonprofessionals who usually described events in their own families. Some of these books were discussed in greater detail by Amy Baker in an article, "The Power of Stories / Stories about Power." Baker said, "This paper outlines the rationale for why reading true and fictional accounts of parental alienation syndrome may be beneficial for parents targeted for PAS. Four true stories are reviewed in detail and several crosscutting themes are identified" (Baker, 2006a). Some of these books–such as *Ex-Etiquette for Parents* and *The Complete Idiot's Guide to Surviving Divorce*–deal with the broad topic of divorced parents and discuss parental alienation in a limited manner. Of course, there have been many books about parental alienation and PAS written by mental health professionals, and they are discussed elsewhere in this book. The following books are listed alphabetically by author.

The Parentectomy: An Individual Perspective on Rising above Parental Alienation, by Kimber Adams (2009).

A Promise to Ourselves: A Journey through Fatherhood and Divorce, by Alec Baldwin and Mark Tabb (2008).

Ex-etiquette for Parents: Good Behavior after a Divorce or Separation, by Jann Blackstone-Ford and Sharyl Jupe (2004).

Lost Children: A Guide for Separating Parents, by Penny Cross (2000).

The Look of Love, by Jill Egizii (2010).

Hilary's Trial: The Elizabeth Morgan Case: A Child's Ordeal in America's Legal System, by Jonathan Groner (1991).

Liebe Mama, Böser Papa: Eltern-Kind-Entfremdung nach Trennung und Scheidung: Das PAS-Syndrom (Dear Mom, Bad Dad: Parent-Child Alienation after Separation and Divorce: The PAS Syndrome) (German), by Gabriele ten Hövel (2003).

A Family's Heartbreak: A Parent's Introduction to Parental Alienation, by Mike Jeffries and Joel Davies (2009).

A Family Divided: A Divorced Father's Struggle with the Child Custody Industry, by Robert Mendelson (1998).

They Are My Children Too: A Mother's Struggle for her Sons, by Catherine L. Meyer and Sally Quinn (1999).

A Kidnapped Mind: A Mother's Heartbreaking Memoir of Parental Alienation, by Pamela Richardson (2006).

Vergiss, dass es Dein Vater ist! Ehemals entfremdete Kinder im Gespräch (Remember That It Is Your Father! Formerly Alienated Children in Conversation) (German), edited by Elisabeth Schmidt and Allard Mees (2006).

Unlawful Flight: A Parental Kidnapping, by Glen C. Schulz (2007).

Perilous Journey: A Mother's International Quest to Rescue her Children–A True Story, by Patricia Sutherland (2002).

The Complete Idiot's Guide to Surviving Divorce, by Pamela Weintraub and Terry Hillman (2005).

Verpasseerd ouderschap (Parenting Broken by PAS) (Dutch), edited by Joep Zander (2009).

FILMS, TELEVISION, AND RADIO

The general public was the intended audience for the following motion pictures, prime-time television shows, and radio programs. These media products–which are representative, not comprehensive–are listed in chronological order.

Fourteen Hours (Twentieth Century-Fox Film Corporation, 1951), directed by Henry Hathaway, featured a suicidal young man who apparently had psychiatric problems because of parental alienation.

Victims of Another War: The Aftermath of Parental Alienation (Parents and Abducted Children Together [PACT], 2004) was a groundbreaking study into the psychology of adults whose childhood was stolen from them due to parental alienation.

"Secrets and Lies" (*NBC News,* October 22, 2004) was a news report regarding parental alienation.

"L'aliénation parentale" ("Parental Alienation") (Radio Notre Dame, *Le Bistrot de la Vie,* August 2005) featured a debate regarding parental alienation in France.

"Eye Opener–Parental Alienation Syndrome" (*The Paula Zahn Show,* CNN, June 19, 2006) was a news report regarding parental alienation.

Jake's Closet (Vanguard Cinema, 2007) explored the mind and experiences of a little boy under the stress of a fractured family.

"Le syndrome d'aliénation parental" ("Parental Alienation Syndrome") (*Les Maternelles,* France 5, January 2007) was a news report concerning parental alienation in France.

"Parental Alienation Syndrome" (*The Gregory Mantell Show,* March 22, 2007) was a television talk show featuring family members affected by parental alienation and experts discussing this topic.

"L'aliénation parentale" ("Parental Alienation") (*Radio Vivre FM,* January 2008) was a radio talk show regarding parental alienation in France.

"L'aliénation parentale" ("Parental Alienation") (*Parenthèse Radio,* March 2008) was a professional debate regarding parental alienation in France.

"Les Enfants du Divorce" ("Children of Divorce") (French) (*C'est la Vie en Plus,* a popular television show about societal problems in Belgium, March 12, 2008) featured several adolescents who talked about their experiences as victims of parental alienation. Part of this show can be seen in French at *http://jaime-papa-et-maman.skynetblogs.be.*

"Brainwashed by My Parents" (*The Dr. Phil Show,* October 3, 2008) was a television talk show featuring family members affected by parental alienation and experts discussing this topic.

A network news program (*The Morning Show with Mike and Juliet,* Fox, December 31, 2008) featured a debate regarding parental alienation.

A Morte Inventada (Fading Away) (Portuguese) (Caraminhola Productions, 2009) was a Brazilian documentary regarding parental alienation.

"C'est aussi mon enfant aussi" ("It's my child, too") (*Planet Justice,* TV France 5, March 2009) was a news report by Nathalie Kaas regarding several children and their parents who have suffered from parental alienation.

"L'aliénation parentale" ("Parental Alienation") (*Le Magasine de la Santé,* TV France 5, March 2009) featured a presentation by professionals regarding parental alienation.

"Rapt parental, et après?" ("Parental kidnapping, and then?) (TF1, *Le Mag,* April 2009) was a news report regarding child abduction and parental alienation.

A network news program in Canada (*W5 Investigates,* CTV News, November 19, 2009) featured the story of Pamela Richardson and the death of her son, Dash.

ORGANIZATIONS AND WEBSITES

The following list of organizations and their Internet websites demonstrates the extent to which the issues of parental alienation and PAS have permeated the popular culture. Although twelve countries are represented in this list, this is only a partial list of organizations and websites devoted to parental alienation and PAS.

A Child's Right: An organization dedicated to a child's fundamental right to be loved, guided, nurtured, and educated by both fit and willing parents (*www.achildsright.typepad.com*).

Associação de Pais e Mães Separados (APASE) (Association of Separated Parents): This Brazilian organization provides information about parental alienation and many other topics (*www.apase.org.br*).

Asociación de Padres Alejados de sus Hijos (APADESHI) (Association of Parents Separated from their Children): This Argentine organization pertains to "dads, moms, grandparents, uncles, new partners in defense of the bond of children with both parents (*www.apadeshi.org.ar*).

Asociación Nacional de Afectados del Síndrome de Alienación Parental (ANASAP) (National Association for Those Affected by Parental Alienation Syndrome): This Argentine organization describes itself as the first national association concerned with the serious mental health problem of parental alienation (*www.anasap.org*).

Association Contre l'Aliénation Parentale (ACALPA): This French organization is devoted to parental alienation (*www.acalpa.org*). Several videos related to the work of ACALPA are located at *www.dailymotion.com/ACALPA.* ACALPA is a nonprofit French organization that promotes awareness and education regarding parental alienation, offers help to parents who have been rejected by their children as a result of PAS, and provides training courses for professionals and gendarmerie officers.

Associazione di Associazioni Nazionali per la Tutela dei Minori (ADIANTUM) (Association of National Associations for the Protection of Minors): This Italian organization seeks to improve the effectiveness of child protection and safeguard children's rights. Their website addresses the problem of parental alienation (*www.adiantum.it*).

Bienvenue sur le site SEPARATION: This is a Belgian website devoted to parental alienation (*www.separation.be*).

Children Need Both Parents, Inc.: This nonprofit organization emphasizes the importance of having two parents in the lives of children (*www.cnbpinc.org*).

Children Rights Council (CRC): This organization works to assure a child the frequent, meaningful, and continuing contact with two parents and extended family after divorce or separation (*www.crckids.org*).

Fathers & Families: This organization seeks to improve the lives of children by protecting the child's right to the love and care of both parents after separation or divorce (*www.fathersandfamilies.org*).

Families Need Fathers: This English organization seeks to obtain the best possible blend of both parents in the lives of their children (*www.fnf.org.uk*).

Gescheiden Ouders Dientsbetoon door Informatie (GOUDI) (Information Site for Divorced Parents): This multilingual European website provides information regarding parental alienation and other topics for divorced parents (*www.goudi.be*).

Japan Children's Rights Network: Their website says, "Our Mission is to disseminate information to help change attitudes and laws in Japan in order to assure all children of direct, meaningful and continuing contact with both parents, regardless of citizenship, marital status or gender" (*www.crnjapan.net*).

Jewish Unity for Multiple Parenting (JUMP): This English organization campaigns for improved relationships between divorced parents and their children in the Jewish community (*www.jump-parenting.org.uk*).

Lee PAS Foundation: This organization was established to promote awareness and education regarding parental alienation, PAS, and parental kidnapping (*www.leepasfoundation.org*).

Life on the Run: My Post-Abduction Diary: The author of this blog is an adult survivor of parental alienation. She was born in Norway and abducted by her father to the U.S. (*http://lifeontherunmypost-abductiondiary.blogspot.com*).

Mothers Apart from Their Children (MATCH): This organization supports mothers after their children have been taken into care, adopted, fostered, abducted abroad, or alienated from them after high-conflict divorce (*www.matchmothers.org/index.html*).

Parental Alienation Awareness Organization (PAAO): This organization seeks to raise awareness of parental alienation and the problems of hostile aggressive parenting (*www.parental-alienation-awareness.com*).

Parental Alienation Awareness Organization–United States (PAAO-US): This organization provides information, stories, and resources related to parental alienation (*www.paao-us.com*).

Parental Alienation Disorder: This website—organized by Ms. Monika Logan, a social worker—provides support and resources for both parents and professionals (*www.parentalalienationsupport.com*).

Parental Alienation Hurts: This website lists blogs, links, and resources (*www.parentalalienationhurts.com*). Its founder, Ms. Chrissy Chrzanowski, was an alienated child who is now an adult, full-time advocate regarding parental alienation.

Parental Alienation Syndrome: This is an Australian website devoted to parental alienation and dedicated to educating people about the devastating effects of parental alienation (*www.parentalalienationcrisis.org*).

PAS-Eltern e.V.: This is a German website devoted to parental alienation (*www.pas-eltern.de*).

Pertubuhan Memupuk Asas Ikatan Keluarga (Basic Organization of Foster Families Association): This is a Malaysian website devoted to parental alienation and fostering family ties (*www.pemalik.org*).

Prevent Parental Kidnap: The goal of this website is to inform, from the child's point of view, the destructive outcomes and abuse from parental kidnapping—a severe form of parental alienation (*www.preventparentalkidnap.org*).

Psychologie & Familienrecht (Psychology and Family Law): This German website has information about parental alienation and related topics (*www.orbation.de*).

Schutzraum eSK: This is a German website devoted to parental alienation (*www.eskhilfe.de.vu*).

Síndrome da Alienação Parental: This is a Brazilian website devoted to parental alienation (*www.alienacaoparental.com.br*).

Split n Two: This website is a place for families and professionals to learn about the devastating effects of parental alienation (*www.splitntwo.org*).

Spravedlnost d_tem (Justice for Children): This is a Czech website devoted to parental alienation and related problems, which offers help to parents who have been rejected by their children as a result of PAS (*www.iustin.cz*).

SOS Papá Asociación pro Derechos del Niño (Association for the Rights of the Child): This organization has organized international conferences in Spain regarding parental alienation (*www.sospapa.es*).

SOS Papai e Mamãe!—União Nacional: This website represents the Association for the Defense and the Study of Equal Paternal, Maternal, and Filial Rights in Brazil (*www.sos-papai.org/en_oque_ap.html*).

Take Root: The website is devoted to child abduction, particularly abduction by family members, which almost always involves parental alienation (*www.takeroot.org*).

The Rachel Foundation for Family Reintegration: This organization provides reintegration programs for parents and children whose bonds of affection have been damaged or destroyed by abduction and/or alienation (*www.*

rachelfoundation.org).

Three Sides to Every Story Inc.: This organization encourages families to take a look at all the possible sides of their situation when children are involved and divorce seems to be the only option (*www.three-sides-to-every-story.org*).

INTERNET SUPPORT GROUPS AND SOCIAL NETWORKING

The following organizations and websites provide support and guidance for parents who have been affected by parental alienation. This is a very limited partial list of support groups and e-groups related to parental alienation and PAS. On Facebook, the social networking website, there are approximately 100 groups representing thousands of parents and extended family members dealing with parental alienation. Yahoo! Groups lists almost 200 e-groups related to these topics. Also, face-to-face support groups have been organized in many cities in the U.S.

Acalpa-Mundi: This is a global social network focused on parental alienation, which is associated with ACALPA, a French advocacy organization (*http://fr-fr.facebook.com/people/Acalpa-Mundi/100000264882453*).

Dads in Action: This is the largest Canadian e-group for fathers who are victims of parental alienation (*http://groups.yahoo.com/group/Dads_In_Action/summary*).

PAS 2000: This is a global e-group focused on parental alienation (*http://groups.yahoo.com/group/PAS2000/summary*).

PAS2ndWivesClub: This is an e-group focused on parental alienation support (*http://groups.yahoo.com/group/PAS2ndWivesClub/summary*).

PAS Parents: This e-group offers support to parents alienated from their children (*http://www.rachelfoundation.org/supportgroup.htm*).

Parents Against Parental Alienation (PAPA): This is an e-group and monthly support group in the United States (*http://groups.yahoo.com/group/ParentsAgainstParentalAlienation/summary*).

INTERNATIONAL PARENTAL ALIENATON AWARENESS DAY

The Parental Alienation Awareness Organization (PAAO), based in Toronto, Ontario, strives to promote education and awareness of parental alienation and the harm it does to children's emotional and mental health. Several years ago, PAAO created International Parental Alienation Awareness Day, which occurs on April 25. (More information is available at *www.paawarenessday.com*.)

By 2009, official proclamations honoring this day were signed by the governors of 15 of the United States: Alabama, Arkansas, Connecticut, Florida, Georgia, Indiana, Iowa, Kentucky, Maine, Maryland, Mississippi, Montana, Nebraska, Nevada, and West Virginia. According to PAAO, these Parental Alienation Proclamations acknowledge the existence of parental alienation within the community and that parental alienation is a severe form of child abuse. Also, on International Parental Alienation Awareness Day, sponsored events have occurred in Austria, Australia, Belgium, Bermuda, Brazil, Canada, the Czech Republic, England, Germany, Italy, Mexico, Poland, Singapore, South Africa, the United Kingdom, and the United States.

Appendix E

BIBLIOGRAPHY REGARDING
PARENTAL ALIENATION

The published works cited in this book are included in the following bibliography. However, this bibliography also includes hundreds of books, book chapters, and papers published in mental health and legal professional journals that were not cited in the text of this book. Most of these references pertain directly to parental alienation or PAS. However, some of these references do not, but they are included here because they pertain to closely-related topics such as domestic violence, child abuse, and research methodology. The international scope of this bibliography is reflected in references from Argentina, Australia, Austria, Belgium, Brazil, Canada, Chile, Cuba, the Czech Republic, Denmark, Finland, France, Germany, India, Israel, Italy, Japan, Latvia, Malaysia, Mexico, the Netherlands, Norway, Poland, Portugal, South Africa, Spain, Sweden, Switzerland, the United Kingdom, and the United States.

Altogether, this bibliography includes more than 630 references. We believe this is the largest bibliography ever developed regarding parental alienation. It includes more than 200 books and book chapters that relate directly to parental alienation or a closely related topic, such as divorce and child custody. The bibliography includes more than 300 articles from professional journals that relate directly to parental alienation or a closely-related topic. In developing this bibliography, we were surprised to locate about 25 doctoral theses regarding parental alienation from universities in Austria, Brazil, Canada, France, Germany, Italy, Spain, Switzerland, and the United States. We believe this reflects a widespread interest in this topic among scholars.

Adams, Kimber (2009). *The parentectomy: An individual perspective on rising above parental alienation.* Bloomington, Indiana: Xlibris Publishing.
Aguilar, José M. (2004). *S.A.P.: Síndrome de Alienación Parental [PAS: Parental*

Alienation Syndrome] [Spanish]. Córdoba, Spain: Almuzara.

Aguilar, José M. (2005). El uso de los hijos en los procesos de separación: El Síndrome de Alienación Parental [The use of children in separation processes: The Parental Alienation Syndrome] [Spanish]. *Revista de Derecho de Familia, 29*(October-December 2005):71–82.

Aguilar, José M. (2007). Interferencias de las relaciones paterno filiales. El Síndrome de Alienación Parental y las nuevas formas de violencia contra la infancia [Interference of the parent-child relationships. Parental alienation syndrome and new forms of violence against children] [Spanish]. *Revista Psicología Educativa, 13*(2):101–16.

Aguilar, José M. (2008a). *Tenemos que hablar [We Need to Talk]* [Spanish]. Madrid: Santillana Ediciones Generales.

Aguilar, José M. (2008b). *Síndrome de Alienaçào Parental [Parental Alienation Syndrome]* [Portuguese]. Lisbon: Caleidoscopio.

Ainsworth, Mary D., Mary C. Blehar, Everett Waters, and Sally Wall. (1978). *Patterns on attachment: A psychological study of the strange situation.* Hillsdale, New Jersey: Lawrence Erlbaum.

Amato, Paul R. (1994). Life-span adjustment of children to their parents' divorce. *Future of Children 4*(1):143–64.

American Academy of Child and Adolescent Psychiatry. (1997a). Practice parameters for the forensic evaluation of children and adolescents who may have been physically or sexually abused. *Journal of the American Academy of Child and Adolescent Psychiatry, 36*(3):423–42.

American Academy of Child and Adolescent Psychiatry. (1997b). Practice parameters for child custody evaluation. *Journal of the American Academy of Child and Adolescent Psychiatry, 36*(10 Suppl):57S–68S.

American Bar Association. (2008). *A judge's guide: Making child-centered decisions in custody cases* (2nd ed.). Chicago, Illinois: American Bar Association.

American Psychiatric Association. (2000). *Diagnostic and statistical manual of mental disorders* (4th ed.). Text Revision. Arlington, Virginia: American Psychiatric Association.

American Psychological Association. (1994). Guidelines for child custody evaluations in divorce proceedings. *American Psychologist, 49*(4):677–80.

American Psychological Association. (1996). Report of the American Psychological Presidential Task Force on Violence and the Family. Washington, D.C.: American Psychological Association.

American Psychological Association. (2005). Women's Psych-E. *www.apa.org,* accessed September 26, 2009.

American Psychological Association. (2008). Statement on Parental Alienation Syndrome. *www.apa.org,* accessed September 26, 2009.

American Psychological Association. (2009). Guidelines for Child Custody Evaluations in Family Law Proceedings. Washington, D.C.: American Psychological Association.

Andre, Katherine C. (2004). Parent alienation syndrome. *Annals of the American Psychotherapy Association, 7*(4):7–11.

Andre, Katherine C., and Amy J. L. Baker. (2009). *I don't want to choose: How middle school kids can avoid choosing one parent over the other.* New York: The Vincent J. Fontana Center for Child Protection.

Andritzky, Walter. (2002a). Verhaltensmuster und Persönlichkeitsstruktur entfremdender Eltern: Psychosoziale Diagnostik und Orientierungskriterien für Interventionen [Behavioral patterns and personality structure of alienating parents: Psychosocial and diagnostic criteria for intervention] [German]. *Psychotherapie in Psychiatrie, Psychotherapeutischer Medizin und Klinischer Psychologie,* 7(2):166–82.

Andritzky, Walter. (2002b). Zur Problematik kinderärztlicher Atteste bei Umgangs- und Sorgerechtsstreitigkeiten I [Concerning problems with pediatric reports in the context of visitation- and custody litigation I] [German]. *Kinder- und Jugendarzt,* 33(11):885–89.

Andritzky, Walter. (2002c). Zur Problematik kinderärztlicher Atteste bei Umgangs- und Sorgerechtsstreitigkeiten II [Concerning problems with pediatric reports in the context of visitation- and custody litigation II] [German]. *Kinder- und Jugendarzt,* 33(12):984–90.

Andritzky, Walter. (2003a). Parental alienation syndrome. *Deutsches Ärzteblatt,* 100(2):81–82.

Andritzky, Walter. (2003b). Kinderpsychiatrische Atteste im Umgangs- und Sorgerechtsstreit–Ergebnisse einer Befragung [Medical letters of child psychiatrists, and their role in custody and visitation litigation–Results of an inquiry] [German]. *Praxis der Kinderpsychologie und Kinderpsychiatrie, 52*(10):794–811.

Andritzky, Walter. (2003c). Entfremdungsstrategien im Sorgerechts- und Umgangsstreit: Zur Rolle von (kinder)ärzlichen und -psychiatrischen "Attesten" [Alienation strategies in custody and visitation litigations: The role of pediatricians', physicians' and psychiatrists' certificates] [German]. In: *Das Parental Alienation Syndrom: Eine interdisziplinäre Herausforderung für scheidungsbegleitende Berufe,* Eds. Wilfrid von Boch-Galhau et al., pages 249–82. Berlin: Verlag für Wissenschaft und Bildung.

Andritzky, Walter. (2003d). Behavioral patterns and personality structure of alienating parents: Psychosocial diagnostic and orientation criteria for intervention. In: *Das Parental Alienation Syndrom: Eine interdisziplinäre Herausforderung für scheidungsbegleitende Berufe,* Eds. Wilfrid von Boch-Galhau et al., pages 283–314. Berlin: Verlag für Wissenschaft und Bildung.

Andritzky, Walter. (2006). The role of medical reports in the development of parental alienation syndrome. In Richard A. Gardner, Demosthenes Lorandos, and S. Richard Sauber (Eds.), *The International Handbook of Parental Alienation Syndrome: Conceptual, Clinical and Legal Considerations,* pages 195–208. Springfield, Illinois: Charles C Thomas.

Anthony, E. James, and Therese Benedek, Eds. (1970). *Parenthood: Its psychology and psychopathology.* Boston: Little, Brown and Company.

Associação de Pais e Mães Separados. (2008). *Síndrome de Alienaçào Parental [Parental Alienation Syndrome]* [Portuguese]. Porto Alegre, Brazil: Editora Equilíbrio.

Association of Family and Conciliation Courts (AFCC) Task Force on Parenting

Coordination. (2006). Guidelines for parenting coordination. *Family Court Review, 44:*164–81.

Austin, Jr. Richard B. (2006). PAS as a child against self. In Richard A. Gardner, S. Richard Sauber, and Demosthenes Lorandos (Eds.), *The International Handbook of Parental Alienation Syndrome: Conceptual, Clinical and Legal Considerations,* pages 56–64. Springfield, Illinois: Charles C Thomas.

Babbie, Earl R. (2007). *The practice of social research* (11th ed.). Florence, Kentucky: Cengage Learning.

Bakalář, Eduard. (1998). Das "Parental Alienation Syndrome" (PAS) in der Tschechischen Republik [The "Parental Alienation Syndrome" (PAS) in the Czech Republic] [German]. *Zentralblatt für Jugendrecht, 85*(6):268.

Bakalář, Eduard. (2002). Syndrom zavrženého rodiče v České republice [Parental alienation syndrome in the Czech Republic] [Czech]. In: *Průvodce otcovstvím, aneb bez otce se nedá (dobre) žít [A Guide through Fatherhood: One Cannot Live Well Without a Father],* pages 109–20. Prague: Vysehrad.

Bakalář, Eduard. (2003). Syndrom zavrženého rodiče [Parental Alienation Syndrome] [Czech]. *Psychologie dnes, 9*(1):28–29.

Bakalář, Eduard. (2006a). What motivates parents to indoctrinate their children with parental alienation syndrome? A perspective from the Czech Republic. In Richard A. Gardner, S. Richard Sauber, and Demosthenes Lorandos (Eds.), *The international handbook of parental alienation syndrome: Conceptual, clinical and legal considerations,* pages 302–09. Springfield, Illinois: Charles C Thomas.

Bakalář, Eduard. (2006b). Syndrom zavržení rodiče. Příčiny, diagnóza, terapie [Parental Alienation Syndrome: Etiology, Diagnostics, Therapy] [Czech]. In: *Rozvodová tematika a moderní psychologie [Divorce Topics and Modern Psychology],* pages 40–58. Prague: Karolinum.

Bakalář, Eduard, and Daniel Novák. (1996). Popouzení dítěte proti druhému rodiči [Inciting the child against the other parent] [Czech]. In: *Průvodce Rozvodem [A Guide Through Divorce],* pages 133–42. Prague: Lidové noviny.

Bakalář, Eduard, and Daniel Novák. (1999). Syndrom zavrženého rodiče v České republice [PAS in the Czech Republic] [Czech]. *Rodinné právo (4):*11–16.

Baker, Amy J. L. (2005a). The long-term effects of parental alienation on adult children: A qualitative research study. *American Journal of Family Therapy, 33*(4):289–302.

Baker, Amy J. L. (2005b). The cult of parenthood: A qualitative study of parental alienation. *Cultic Studies Review, 4*(1):np.

Baker, Amy J. L. (2005c). Parent alienation strategies: A qualitative study of adults who experienced parental alienation as a child. *American Journal of Forensic Psychology, 23*(4):41–63.

Baker, Amy J. L. (2006a). The power of stories/stories about power: Why therapists and clients should read stories about the parental alienation syndrome. *American Journal of Family Therapy, 34*(3):191–203.

Baker, Amy J. L. (2006b). Patterns of parental alienation syndrome: A qualitative study of adults who were alienated from a parent as a child. *American Journal of Family Therapy, 34*(1):63–78.

Baker, Amy J. L. (2007a). Knowledge and attitudes about the parental alienation syndrome: A survey of custody evaluators. *American Journal of Family Therapy, 35*(1):1–19.

Baker, Amy J. L. (2007b). *Adult children of parental alienation syndrome: Breaking the ties that bind.* New York: W. W. Norton & Co.

Baker, Amy J. L. (2010). Adult recall of parental alienation in a community sample: Prevalence and associations with psychological maltreatment. *Journal of Divorce & Remarriage, 51*(1):16–35.

Baker, Amy J. L., and Katherine Andre (2008). Working with alienated children and their targeted parents. *Annals of the American Psychotherapy Association, 11*(2):10–17.

Baker, Amy J. L., and Douglas Darnall. (2006). Behaviors and strategies employed in parental alienation: A survey of parental experiences. *Journal of Divorce & Remarriage, 45*(1–2):97–124.

Baker, Amy J. L., and Douglas Darnall. (2007). A construct study of the eight symptoms of severe parental alienation syndrome: A survey of parental experiences. *Journal of Divorce & Remarriage, 47*(1–2):55–75.

Baldwin, Alec, and Mark Tabb. (2008). *A promise to ourselves: A journey through fatherhood and divorce.* New York: St. Martin's Press.

Barber, Brian K. (1996). Parental psychological control: Revisiting a neglected construct. *Child Development, 67*(6):(3)296–319.

Barden, R. Christopher. (2003). Building multi-disciplinary legal-scientific teams in PAS and child custody cases. In: *Das Parental Alienation Syndrom: Eine interdisziplinäre Herausforderung für scheidungsbegleitende Berufe,* Eds. Wilfrid von Boch-Galhau et al., pages 373–81. Berlin: Verlag fur Wissenschaft und Bildung.

Barden, R. Christopher. (2006). Protecting the fundamental rights of children and families: Parental alienation syndrome and family law reform. In Richard A. Gardner, S. Richard Sauber, and Demosthenes Lorandos (Eds.), *The international handbook of parental alienation syndrome: Conceptual, clinical and legal consideration,* pages 419–32. Springfield, Illinois: Charles C Thomas.

Baurain, Martine. (2005). Dossier l'aliénation parentale: Pour poser les termes du débat [Dossier on the parental alienation syndrome: For posing the terms for debate] [French]. *Divorce et Séparation,* (3):5–12.

Bäuerle, Siegfried and Helgard Moll-Strobel, Eds. (2001). *Eltern sägen ihr Kind entzwei −Trennungserfahrungen und Entfremdung von einem Elternteil [Parents Sawing Their Child Apart: Separation Experiences and Alienation of a Parent]* [German]. Donauwörth, Germany: Auer Verlag.

Beach, Steven R. H., Marianne Z. Wamboldt, Nadine J. Kaslow, Richard E. Heyman, and David Reiss. (2006). Relational processes and mental health: A bench-to-bedside dialogue to guide DSM-V. In Steven R. H. Beach et al. (Eds.), *Relational processes and DSM-V: Neuroscience, assessment, prevention, and intervention,* pages 1–18. Washington, DC: American Psychiatric Press.

Beardslee, William R., and Lisbeth A. Hoke. (1997). Children of parents with chronic illness: The effects of parental depression and parental cancer. In: *Handbook of child and adolescent psychiatry,* Vol. 6, Ed. Joseph D. Noshpitz, pages 64–76. New York: John Wiley & Sons.

Beeble, Marisa L., Deborah Bybee, and Cris M. Sullivan. (2007). Abusive men's use of children to control their partners and ex-partners. *European Psychologist, 12*(1):54–61.

Bellerose, Jean-Guy. (1998). De L'Impasse Du Divorce à L'Aliénation Parentale [From a Divorce Deadlock to Parental Alienation] [French]. Dissertation, McGill University, Canada.

Benedek, Elissa P., and Diane H. Schetky. (1985a). Allegations of sexual abuse in child custody and visitation disputes. In Elissa P. Benedek and Diane H. Schetky (Eds.), *Emerging issues in child psychiatry and the law,* pages 145–56. New York: Brunner/Mazel.

Benedek, Elissa P., and Diane H. Schetky. (1985b). Custody and visitation: Problems and perspectives. *Psychiatric Clinics of North America, 8*(4):857–873.

Benedek, Elissa P., and Diane H. Schetky. (1987a). Problems in validating allegations of sexual abuse. Part 1: Factors affecting perception and recall of events. *Journal of the American Academy of Child and Adolescent Psychiatry, 26*(6):912–15.

Benedek, Elissa P., and Diane H. Schetky (1987b). Problems in validating allegations of sexual abuse. Part 2: Clinical Evaluation. *Journal of the American Academy of Child and Adolescent Psychiatry, 26*(6):916–21.

Bensussan, Paul. (1999). *Inceste, le piège du soupçon [Incest, the Trap of Suspicion]* [French]. Paris: Editions Belfond.

Bensussan, Paul. (2005). Interview du Docteur Paul Bensussan [Interview of Doctor Paul Bensussan] [French]. *Divorce et Séparation,* (3):78–89.

Bensussan, Paul. (2009). L'aliénation parentale: vers la fin du déni? [Parental alienation: Toward the end of the denial?] [French]. *Annales Médico-Psychologiques,* (167):409–15.

Bensussan, Paul, and Florence Rault. (2002). *La Dictature de l'émotion: La Protection de l'enfant et ses dérives [The Dictate of Emotions: The Protection of the Child and its Tendencies]* [French]. Paris: Editions Belfond.

Bergman, Z. B., and E. Weitzman. (1995). Parental kidnapping and parental alienation. *Sichot, 9*(2):115–30.

Bernet, William (1993). False statements and the differential diagnosis of abuse allegations. *Journal of the American Academy of Child and Adolescent Psychiatry,* 32(5):903–10.

Bernet, William. (1995). *Children of divorce: A practical guide for parents, attorneys, and therapists.* New York: Vantage.

Bernet, William. (1997). Case study: Allegations of abuse created in a single interview. *Journal of the American Academy of Child and Adolescent Psychiatry, 36*(7):966–70.

Bernet, William. (1998). The child and adolescent psychiatrist and the law. In Joseph D. Noshpitz (Ed.), *Handbook of Child and Adolescent Psychiatry,* Vol. 7, pages 438–67. New York: John Wiley & Sons.

Bernet, William. (2002). Child custody evaluations. *Child and Adolescent Psychiatric Clinics of North America, 11*(4):781–804.

Bernet, William. (2006). Sexual abuse allegations in the context of child custody disputes. In Richard A. Gardner, S. Richard Sauber, and Demosthenes Lorandos (Eds.), *The international handbook of parental alienation syndrome: Conceptual, clinical*

Boch-Galhau, Wilfrid von, Ursula Kodjoe, Walter Andritzky, and Peter Koeppel, Eds. (2003). *Das Parental Alienation Syndrom: Eine interdisziplinäre Herausforderung für scheidungsbegleitende Berufe [The Parental Alienation Syndrome: An Interdisciplinary Challenge for Professionals Involved with Divorce]* [German]. Berlin: Verlag für Wissenschaft und Bildung.

Bolaños Cartujo, José Ignacio. (2000). Estudio Descriptivo Del Síndrome De Alienación Parental En Procesos De Separación y Divorcio. Diseño y Aplicación De Un Programa Piloto De Mediación Familiar [Descriptive Study of the Parental Alienation Syndrome in the Course of Separation and Divorce. Design and Application of a Pilot Program in Family Mediation] [Spanish]. Unpublished doctoral dissertation, Universitat Autónoma de Barcelona, Barcelona.

Bolaños Cartujo, José Ignacio. (2002). El síndrome de alienación parental. Descripción y abordajes psico-legales [The parental alienation syndrome. Description and psycho-legal approaches] [Spanish]. *Psicopatología Clínica Legal y Forense, 2*(3):25–45.

Bolaños Cartujo, José Ignacio. (2008). *Hijos alineados y padres alienados. Mediación familiar en rupturas conflictivas [Aligned Children and Alienated Parents. Family Mediation in Conflictual Separations]* [Spanish]. Madrid: Reus.

Bolaños Cartujo, José Ignacio. (2009). Del Síndrome de Alienación Parental al Síndrome de Alienación Familiar a través de una Mediación Transicional [From Parental Alienation Syndrome to Family Alienation Syndrome through a Transitional Mediation] [Spanish]. *Proyecto Hombre,* (66):36–39.

Bond, Richard. (2007). The lingering debate over the parental alienation syndrome phenomenon. *Journal of Child Custody, 4*(1–2):37–54.

Bone, J. Michael. (2003). The parental alienation syndrome: Examing the validity amid controversy. *Family Law Section Commentator, 20*(1):24–27.

Bone, J. Michael, and Michael R. Walsh. (1999). Parental alienation syndrome: How to detect it and what to do about it. *Florida Bar Journal, 73*(3):44–47.

Borris, Edward B. (1997). Interference with parental rights of noncustodial parent as grounds for modification of child custody. *Divorce Litigation, 8*:1–13.

Bouchard, Thomas J., Jr. (1976). Unobtrusive measures: An inventory of uses. *Sociological Methods and Research, 4*:267–300.

Bow, James N., Jonathan W. Gould, and James R. Flens. (2009). Examining parental alienation in child custody cases: A survey of mental health and legal professionals. *American Journal of Family Therapy, 37*(2):127–45.

Bowen, Murray. (1966). The use of family theory in clinical practice. *Comprehensive Psychiatry, 7*:345–74.

Bowen, Murray. (1978). *Family therapy in clinical practice.* Northvale, N.J.: Jason Aronson.

Bowlby, John. (1988). *A secure base: Clinical applications of attachment theory.* London: Routledge.

Brandes, Joel R. (2000). Parental alienation. *New York Law Journal,* (March 26).

Bricklin, Barry. (1984). *Bricklin Perceptual Scales.* Furlong, Pennsylvania: Village Publishing.

Bricklin, Barry. (1990). *PORT Handbook: Perception-of-Relationships-Test.* Doylestown,

Pennsylvania: Village Publishing.

Bricklin, Barry. (1995). *The custody evaluation handbook: Research-based solutions and applications.* New York: Brunner/Mazel.

Bricklin, Barry, and Gail Elliot. (2002). *The Perception-of-Relationships-Test (PORT) and Bricklin Perceptual Scales (BPS): Current and new empirical data on 3,880 cases, 1961–2002.* Furlong, Pennsylvania: Village Publishing.

Bricklin, Barry, and Gail Elliot. (2006). Psychological test-assisted detection of parental alienation syndrome. In Richard A. Gardner, S. Richard Sauber, and Demosthenes Lorandos (Eds.), *The international handbook of parental alienation syndrome: Conceptual, clinical and legal consideration,* pages 264–75. Springfield, Illinois: Charles C Thomas.

Brock, Michael G., and Samuel Saks. (2008). *Contemporary issues in family law and mental health.* Springfield, Illinois: Charles C Thomas.

Brody, Barry. (2006a). The misdiagnosis of PAS. In Richard A. Gardner, S. Richard Sauber, and Demosthenes Lorandos (Eds.), *The international handbook of parental alienation syndrome: Conceptual, clinical and legal consideration,* pages 209–27. Springfield, Illinois: Charles C Thomas.

Brody, Barry. (2006b). Criticism of PAS in courts of law: How to deal with it and why it occurs. In Richard A. Gardner, S. Richard Sauber, and Demosthenes Lorandos (Eds.), *The international handbook of parental alienation syndrome: Conceptual, clinical and legal consideration,* pages 372–77. Springfield, Illinois: Charles C Thomas.

Brögger, Jan. (1995). Når barn utvikler sykelig hat mot foreldre [When children develop morbid hatred toward parents] [Norwegian]. *Aftenposten,* January 21, 1995.

Brown, Carole. (1993). The impact of divorce on families: The Australian experience. *Family & Conciliation Courts Review, 2*:149–67.

Brown, Ron. (2005). Fairshare cases: Competency to enter stipulation; anger management; PAS testimony; pre-marital covenant not to compete. *American Journal of Family Law, 19*(2):143.

Brownstone, Harvey. (2009a). *Tug of war: A judge's verdict on separation, custody battles, and the bitter realities of family court.* Toronto: ECW Press.

Brownstone, Harvey. (2009b). That toxic tug-of-war. *Globe and Mail,* April 24, 2009.

Bruch, Carol S. (2001a). Parental alienation syndrome: Junk science in child custody determinations. *European Journal of Law Reform, 3*:383.

Bruch, Carol S. (2001b). Parental alienation syndrome and parental alienation: Getting it wrong in child custody cases. *Family Law Quarterly, 35*(3):527–52.

Bruch, Carol S. (2002). Parental alienation syndrome and alienated children: Getting it wrong in child custody cases. *Child and Family Law Quarterly, 14*(4):381–400.

Burrill, Janelle. (2001). Parental alienation syndrome in court referred custody cases. Dissertation, Northcentral University, Prescott Valley, Arizona.

Burrill, Janelle. (2006a). Descriptive statistics of the mild, moderate, and severe characteristics of parental alienation syndrome. In Richard A. Gardner, S. Richard Sauber, and Demosthenes Lorandos (Eds.), *The international handbook of parental alienation syndrome: Conceptual, clinical and legal consideration,* pages 49–55. Springfield, Illinois: Charles C Thomas.

Burrill, Janelle. (2006b). Reluctance to verify PAS as a legitimate syndrome. In Richard A. Gardner, S. Richard Sauber, and Demosthenes Lorandos (Eds.), *The international handbook of parental alienation syndrome: Conceptual, clinical and legal consideration,* pages 323–30. Springfield, Illinois: Charles C Thomas.

Buzzi, Isabella. (1997). La Sindrome di Alienazione Genitoriale [Parental alienation syndrome] [Italian]. In: *Separazione, Divorzio e Affidamento dei Figli,* Eds. Vittorio Cigoli, Guglielmo Gulotta, and Giuseppe Santi, pages 177–87. Milan: Giuffré.

Buzzi, Isabella. (2007). La Sindrome di Alienazione Genitoriale [Parental alienation syndrome] [Italian]. In: *Separazione, Divorzio e Affidamento dei Figli,* 2nd ed., Eds. Vittorio Cigoli, Guglielmo Gulotta, and Giuseppe Santi, pages 177–212. Milan: Giuffré.

Byrne, Ken. (1989). Brainwashing in custody cases: The parental alienation syndrome. *Australian Family Lawyer, 4*(3):1–4.

Campbell, Donald T., and Donald W. Fiske. (1959). Convergent and discriminate validation by the multitrait multimethod matrix. *Psychological Bulletin, 56:*81–105.

Campbell, Terence W. (1992a). Psychotherapy with children of divorce: The pitfalls of triangulated relationships. *Psychotherapy: Theory, Research, Practice, and Training, 29.*646–52.

Campbell, Terence W. (1992b). False allegations of sexual abuse and their apparent credibility. *American Journal of Forensic Psychology, 10*(4):21.

Campbell, Terence W. (1993). Parental conflicts between divorced spouses: Strategies for intervention. *Journal of Systemic Therapies, 12*(4):27.

Campbell, Terence W. (2005). Why doesn't parental alienation occur more frequently? The significance of role discrimination. *American Journal of Family Therapy, 33*(5):365–77.

Camps, Astrid. (2003). Psychiatrische und psychosomatische Konsequenzen für PAS-Kinder [Psychiatric and psychosomatic consequences for PAS children] [German]. In: *Das Parental Alienation Syndrom: Eine interdisziplinäre Herausforderung für scheidungsbegleitende Berufe,* Eds. Wilfrid von Boch-Galhau et al., pages 143–55. Berlin: Verlag fur Wissenschaft und Bildung.

Cantón Duarte, José, María del Rosario Cortés Arboleda, and María Dolores Justicia Diaz. (2002). *Conflictos matrimoniales, divorcio y desarrollo de los hijos [Marital Disputes, Divorce and Child Development]* [Spanish]. Madrid: Pirámide.

Carey, Kristen Marie. (2003). Exploring long-term outcomes of the parental alienation syndrome. Dissertation, Alliant International University, San Francisco, California.

Cartié, Mercé, Ramón Casany, Raquel Domínguez, Mercé Gamero, Cristina Garcia, Mati Gonzalez, and Carolina Pastor. (2005). Análisis descriptivo de las características asociadas al síndrome de alienación parental (SAP) [Descriptive analysis of characteristics associated with parental alienation syndrome (PAS)] [Spanish]. *Psicopatología Clínica Legal y Forense, 5*(1–3):5–29.

Cartwright, Glenn F. (1993). Expanding the parameters of parental alienation syndrome. *American Journal of Family Therapy, 21*(3):205–15.

Cartwright, Glenn F. (2006). Beyond parental alienation syndrome: Reconciling the alienated child and the lost parent. In Richard A. Gardner, S. Richard Sauber, and Demosthenes Lorandos (Eds.), *The international handbook of parental alienation syndrome: Conceptual, clinical and legal consideration,* pages 286–91. Springfield, Illinois: Charles C Thomas.

Caspi, Avshalom, and Glen H. Elder. (1988). Emergent family patterns: The inter-generational construction of problem behaviour and relationships. In Robert A. Hinde and Joan Stevenson-Hinde (Eds.), *Relationships within families: Mutual influence,* pages 218–40. New York: Oxford University Press.

Ceci, Stephen J., and Maggie Bruck. (1993). Suggestibility of the child witness: A historical review and synthesis. *Psychological Bulletin, 113*(3):403–39.

Ceci, Stephen J., and Maggie Bruck. (1995). *Jeopardy in the courtroom: A scientific analysis of children's testimony.* Washington, DC: American Psychological Association.

Ceci, Stephen J., and Maggie Bruck. (2006). Children's suggestibility: Characteristics and mechanisms. *Advances in Child Development and Behavior, 34:*247–81.

Ceci, Stephen J., Mary Lyndia Crotteau Huffman, Elliott Smith, and Elizabeth F. Loftus. (1994). Repeatedly thinking about a non-event: Source misattributions among preschoolers. *Consciousness and Cognition, 3*(3/4):388–407.

Cialdini, Robert B. (1985). *Influence: Science and practice.* New York: Allyn & Bacon.

Clawar, Stanley S., and Brynne V. Rivlin. (1991). *Children held hostage: Dealing with programmed and brainwashed children.* Chicago, Illinois: American Bar Association.

Colarossi, Melissa. (2007). The different voices of separation and divorce. Dissertation, Concordia University, Montreal, Quebec.

Cooke, Lisa. (1995). Parental alienation syndrome: A hidden facet of custody disputes. First Place, Lieff Award, Canadian Bar Association, Ottawa, Canada.

Corrêa da Fonseca, Priscila Maria Pereira. (2006). Síndrome de alienação parentale [Parental alienation syndrome] [Portuguese]. *Pediatria (São Paulo), 28*(3):162–68.

Cross, Penny. (2000). *Lost children: A guide for separating parents.* London: Velvet Glove Publishing.

D'Agostino, Lucia. (2007). La Sindrome Di Alienazione Genitoriale e i Casi Di Sospetto Abuso Sessuale Infantile: Un Problema Di Diagnosi [The Parental Alienation Syndrome and Cases of Suspected Child Sexual Abuse: A Problem of Diagnosis] [Italian]. Dissertation, Università degli Studi G. d'Annunzio Chieti Pescara, Italy.

Danielsen, Svend. (2004). *Forældres pligter, börns rettigheder [Parents' Duties, Children's Rights]* [Danish]. Copenhagen: Nordisk Ministerråd.

Darnall, Douglas. (1998). *Divorce casualties: Protecting your children from parental alienation.* Dallas, Texas: Taylor Trade Publishing.

Darnall, Douglas. (1999). Parental alienation: Not in the best interest of the children. *North Dakota Law Review, 75:*323.

Darnall, Douglas. (2008). *Divorce casualties: Understanding parental alienation* (2nd ed.). Lanham, Maryland: National Book Network.

Darnall, Douglas, and Barbara F. Steinberg. (2008a). Motivational models for spontaneous renunciation with the alienated child: Part I. *The American Journal of Family Therapy, 36*(2): 107–115.

Darnall, Douglas, and Barbara F. Steinberg. (2008b). Motivational models for spontaneous renunciation with the alienated child: Part II. *The American Journal of*

Family Therapy, 36(3): 253–261.

Darnall, Douglas. (2010). *Beyond divorce casualties: Reunifying the alienated family.* Lanham, Maryland: Taylor Trade Publishing.

De Becker, Emmanuel, and Nawshad Ali-Hamed. (2006). Les fausses allégations d'abus sexuels sur mineurs d'ége : Entre Munchausen par procuration et aliéna-tion parentale [False allegations of sexual abuse on under aged persons: Between Munchausen by proxy and parental alienation] [French]. *L'Évolution Psychiatrique, 71*(3):471–83.

Deed, Martha L. (1991). Court-ordered custody evaluations: Helping or victimizing vulnerable families. *Psychotherapy: Theory, Research, Practice, and Training, 28*(1): 76–84.

Deegener, Günther, and Wilhelm Körner, Eds. (2005). *Kindesmisshandlung und Vernachlässigung–Ein Handbuch [Child Abuse and Neglect–A Handbook]* [German]. Göttingen: Hogrefe.

Del Pozo, Ana Belén. (2008). Un infierno dentro del hogar [Hell within the home] [Spanish]. *Iuris: Actualidad y práctica del derecho, 131.*6–8.

Delfieu, Jean-Marc. (2005). Syndrome d'aliénation parentale: Diagnostic et prise en charge médico-juridique [Parental alienation syndrome: Diagnosis and medical-legal management] [French]. *Experts, 67.*24–30.

Deming, James. (2001). Book review of *Therapeutic interventions for children with parental alienation syndrome,* by Richard Gardner. *Journal of the American Academy of Psychiatry and the Law, 29*(4):505.

Dennis, Norman, and George Erdos. (1992). *Families without fatherhood.* London: IEA Health & Welfare Unit.

Derdeyn, Andre P. (1976). A consideration of legal issues in child custody contests. *Archives of General Psychiatry, 33:*161–71.

Despert, J. Louise. (1953). *Children of divorce.* New York: Doubleday.

Deters, Jean Andrew. (2003). Parenting coordination services: A forensic interven-tion for high-conflict child custody cases when parental alienation syndrome is present. Dissertation, Spalding University, Louisville, Kentucky.

Dettenborn, Harry. (2001). *Kindeswohl und Kindeswille: Psychologische und rechtliche Aspekte [Best Interest of the Child and Child's Will: Psychological and Legal Aspects]* [German]. München: E. Reinhardt.

Dettenborn, Harry. (2002). Kindeswille und PAS [Child's will and PAS] [German]. In: *Qualitätssicherung in der Rechtspsychologie,* Eds. Thomas Fabian et al., pages 183–97. Münster: Lit-Verlag.

Dettwiler-Bienz, Susanne. (2003). Die Entfremdung des Kindes von einem Elternteil in Scheidungssituationen. Parental Alienation Syndrome / Entstehung und Auswirkung der Entfremdung und Interventionsmöglichkeiten [The Alienation of a Child from a Parent in Divorce Situations. Parental Alienation Syndrome / Development and Effects of Alienation and Possibilities for Intervention] [German]. Dissertation, Fachhochschule Zürich, Switzerland.

Deutsch, Robin, Matthew Sullivan, and Peggy Ward. (2008). Breaking barriers: An innovative program for alienated and estranged children. *AFCC News, 27.*8–9.

Dias, Maria Berenice. (2006). Síndrome da alienação parental, o que é isso? [Parental alienation syndrome, what is it?] [Portuguese]. *Jus Navigandi, 10*(1119) (July 25, 2006). *http://jus2.uol.com.br/doutrina/texto.asp?id=8690,* accessed January 23, 2010.

Dias, Maria Berenice, Ed. (2007). *Incesto e Alienação Parental [Incest and Parental Alienation]* [Portuguese]. São Paulo, Brazil: Revista dos Tribunais.

Dickstein, Leah J. (2005). Relational problems. In: *Comprehensive textbook of psychiatry,* Eds. Benjamin J. Saddock and Virginia A. Saddock, pages 2241–46. Philadelphia: Lippincott Williams & Wilkins.

Dreger, Monika. (2007). Syndrom PAS, czyli rola dziecka w konflikcie okolorozwodowym [PAS syndrome, or the role of the child in divorce conflict] [Polish]. *www.psycholodzy.pl,* accessed February 1, 2010.

Drozd, Leslie M. (2009). Rejection in cases of abuse or alienation in divorcing families. In Robert M. Galatzer-Levy, Louis Kraus, and Jeanne Galatzer-Levy (Eds.), *The scientific basis for child custody decisions.* New York: John Wiley & Sons.

Drozd, Leslie M., and Nancy Williams Olesen. (2004). Is it abuse, alienation, and/or estrangement? A decision tree. *Journal of Child Custody, 1*(3):65–106.

Dum, Christian. (2003). Begutachtete Aufsätze in Fachzeitschriften und das Parental Alienation Syndrome [Peer-reviewed articles in professional journals and the parental alienation syndrome] [German]. In: *Das Parental Alienation Syndrom: Eine interdisziplinäre Herausforderung für scheidungsbegleitende Berufe,* Eds. Wilfrid von Boch-Galhau et al., pages 384–89. Berlin: Verlag für Wissenschaft und Bildung.

Duncan, J. W. (1978). Medical, psychologic, and legal aspects of child custody disputes. *Mayo Clinic Proceedings, 53*(7):463–68.

Dunkley, Christine. (2007). Review of *The international handbook of parental alienation syndrome. British Journal of Guidance & Counselling, 35*(3):357–58.

Dunne, John, and Marsha Hedrick. (1994). The parental alienation syndrome: An analysis of sixteen selected cases. *Journal of Divorce & Remarriage, 21*(3–4):21–38.

Eastman, A. Margaret, and Thomas J. Moran. (1991). Multiple perspectives: Factors related to differential diagnosis of sex abuse and divorce trauma in children under six. *Child & Youth Services, 15*(2):159–76.

Ebert, Kurt. (2003). Die Rechtssituation bei Kindesentfremdung im europäischen Vergleich, dargestellt vornehmlich an Fallbeispielen der Straßburger Menschenrechts-Judikatur [The legal situation in cases of child alienation in a comparison of different European countries, shown by case examples from the Strasbourg Human-Rights Judicature] [German]. In: *Das Parental Alienation Syndrom: Eine interdisziplinäre Herausforderung für scheidungsbegleitende Berufe,* Eds. Wilfrid von Boch-Galhau et al., pages 19–54. Berlin: Verlag für Wissenschaft und Bildung.

Editorial. (2005). PAS testimony allowed under Frye test. *American Journal of Family Law, 19*(2):148.

Egan, Louisa C., Laurie R. Santos, and Paul Bloom. (2007). The origins of cognitive dissonance: Evidence from children and monkeys. *Psychological Science, 18*(11):978–83.

Egizii, Jill. (2009). *The look of love.* Dallas, Texas: Brown Books Publishing Group.

Ellis, Elizabeth M. (2000). *Divorce wars: Interventions with families in conflict.* Washington D.C.: American Psychological Association.

Ellis, Elizabeth M. (2005). Help for the alienated parent. *American Journal of Family Therapy, 33*(5):415–26.

Ellis, Elizabeth M. (2007). A stepwise approach to evaluating children for parental alienation syndrome. *Journal of Child Custody, 4*(1–2):55–78.

Ellis, Elizabeth M. and Boyan, Susan. (in press). Intervention strategies for parent coordinators in parental alienation cases. *American Journal of Family Therapy.*

Emery, Robert E. (2005). Parental alienation syndrome: Proponents bear the burden of proof. *Family Court Review, 43*(1):8–13.

Emtestam, Gösta, and Agnetha Svensson. (2005). *Vårdnads-, boende- och umgänge-sutredningar [Custody-, Residence- and Visitation-investigations]* [Swedish]. Stockholm: Norstedts Juridik.

Erwoine, Didier. (2005). Les traitements du syndrome d'aliénation parentale [The treatment of parental alienation syndrome] [French]. *Divorce et Séparation,* (3):117–25.

Etemad, Jacqueline. (1999). Review of *The parental alienation syndrome. Journal of the American Academy of Child and Adolescent Psychiatry, 38*(2):223–25.

Everett, Craig A. (2006). Family therapy for parental alienation syndrome: Understanding the interlocking pathologies. In Richard A. Gardner, S. Richard Sauber, and Demosthenes Lorandos (Eds.), *The international handbook of parental alienation syndrome: Conceptual, clinical and legal consideration,* pages 228–41. Springfield, Illinois: Charles C Thomas.

Faculty, Judge Advocate General's School. (2002). Family law note: A quick look at parental alienation syndrome. *Army Lawyer* (March 1, 2002).

Falco, Eugene. (2003). Commentary: Children and divorce. *Journal of the American Academy of Psychiatry and the Law, 31*(2):171–72.

Faller, Kathleen Coulborn. (1998). The parental alienation syndrome: What is it and what data support it? *Child Maltreatment, 3*(2):100–15.

Fariña Rivera, Francisca, Dolores Seijo Martínez, Ramón Arce Fernández, and Mercedes Novo Pérez. (2002). *Psicología Jurídica de la Familia. Intervención de casos de Separación y Divorcio [Psychology of Family Law. Intervention in Cases of Separation and Divorce]* [Spanish]. Barcelona: Cedecs.

Festinger, Leon. (1957). *A theory of cognitive dissonance.* Stanford, California: Stanford University Press.

Festinger, Leon, and J. M. Carlsmith. (1959). Cognitive consequences of forced compliance. *Journal of Abnormal and Social Psychology, 58*:203–10.

Fidler, Barbara Jo, and Nicholas Bala. (2010). Children resisting postseparation contact with a parent: Concepts, controversies, and conundrums. *Family Court Review, 48*(1):10–47.

Fidler, Barbara Jo, Nicholas Bala, Rachel Birnbaum, and Katherine Kavassalis. (2008a). Understanding child alienation and its impact on families. In Barbara Jo Fidler et al., *Challenging issues in child custody assessments: A guide for legal and mental health professional,* pages 203–29. Toronto: Thomson Carswell.

Fidler, Barbara Jo, Nicholas Bala, Rachel Birnbaum, and Katherine Kavassalis. (2008b). *Challenging issues in child custody assessments: A guide for legal and mental health professionals.* Toronto: Thomson Carswell.

Fields, Hope, and Erika Rivera Ragland. (2003). Parental alienation syndrome: What professionals need to know, Part 2 of 2. *NCPCA Update Newsletter, 16*(7).

Figdor, Helmuth. (2003). Psychodynamik bei sogenannten "Entfremdungsprozessen" im Erleben von Kindern–Ein kritischer Beitrag zum PAS-Konzept [Psychodynamic aspects in so-called "alienation processes" as experienced by children–A critical contribution to the PAS concept] [German]. In: *Das Parental Alienation Syndrom: Eine interdisziplinäre Herausforderung für scheidungsbegleitende Berufe,* Eds. Wilfrid von Boch-Galhau et al., pages 187–206. Berlin: Verlag für Wissenschaft und Bildung.

Finkelstein, Cecile. (2003). The heart of an abducted and alienated child. Sarah or Cecile: The identity issue. In: *Das Parental Alienation Syndrom: Eine interdisziplinäre Herausforderung für scheidungsbegleitende Berufe,* Eds. Wilfrid von Boch-Galhau et al., pages 175–85. Berlin: Verlag für Wissenschaft und Bildung.

First, Michael B., Carl C. Bell, Bruce Cuthbert, John H. Krystal, Robert Malison, David R. Offord, David Reiss, M. Tracie Shea, Tom Widiger, and Katherine L. Wisner. (2002). Personality disorders and relational disorders. In David J. Kupfer, Michael B. First, and Darrel A. Regier (Eds.), *A research agenda for DSM-V,* pages 123–99. Washington, DC: American Psychiatric Association.

Fischer, Wera. (1998a). The Parental Alienation Syndrome (PAS) und die Interessenvertretung des Kindes–ein kooperatives Interventionsmodell für Jugendhilfe und Gericht, Frankfurt [The parental alienation syndrome (PAS) and the interests of the child–a collaborative intervention model for youth services and courts, Frankfurt] [German]. *Nachrichtendienst des deutschen Vereins für öffentliche und private Fürsorge, 78*(10):306–09.

Fischer, Wera. (1998b). The Parental Alienation Syndrome (PAS) und die Interessenvertretung des Kindes–ein kooperatives Interventionsmodell für Jugendhilfe und Gericht, Frankfurt [The parental alienation syndrome (PAS) and the interests of the child–a collaborative intervention model for youth services and courts, Frankfurt] [German]. *Nachrichtendienst des deutschen Vereins für öffentliche und private Fürsorge, 78*(11):343–48.

Fischer, Wera. (2003). Möglichkeiten von Verfahrenspflegern in der Arbeit mit PAS-Fällen–Grundsätzliche Aspekte [Working strategies with PAS cases for guardians ad litem–Fundamental aspects] [German]. In: *Das Parental Alienation Syndrom: Eine interdisziplinäre Herausforderung für scheidungsbegleitende Berufe,* Eds. Wilfrid von Boch-Galhau et al., pages 315–21. Berlin: Verlag für Wissenschaft und Bildung.

Folberg, Jay. (1991). *Joint custody and shared parenting.* New York: The Guilford Press.

Freckelton, Ian. (2002). Evaluating parental alienation and child sexual abuse accommodation evidence. *Butterworths Family Law Journal, 4*(3):57–66.

Gagné, Marie-Hélène, and Sylvie Drapeau. (2005). L'aliénation parentale est-elle une forme de maltraitance psychologique? [Is parental alienation a form of child abuse?] [French]. *Divorce et Séparation,* (3):29–42.

Gagné, Marie-Hélène, Sylvie Drapeau, and Rosalie Hénault. (2005). Parental alienation: An overview of research and controversy. *Canadian Psychology-Psychologie Canadienne, 46*(2):73–87.

Gagné, Marie-Hélène, Sylvie Drapeau, Claudiane Melançon, Marie-Christine Saint-

Jacques, and Rachel Lépine. (2007). Links between parental psychological violence, other family disturbances, and children's adjustment. *Family Process, 46*(4):523–42.

Gagnon, Stewart W. (1999). How to identify and deal with parental alienation in your family law case. 25th Advanced Family Law Course, Dallas, Texas, August 16–19, 1999.

Galatzer-Levy, Robert M., Louis Kraus, and Jeanne Galatzer-Levy (Eds.). (2009). *The scientific basis for child custody decisions* (2nd ed.). New York: John Wiley & Sons.

Garbarino, James, Edna Guttmann, and Janis Wilson Seeley. (1986). *The psychologically battered child: Strategies for identification, assessment and intervention.* San Francisco: Jossey-Bass.

Garber, Benjamin D. (1996). Alternatives to parental alienation syndrome: Acknowledging the broader scope of children's emotional difficulties during parental separation and divorce. *New Hampshire Bar Journal, 37*(1):51–54.

Garber, Benjamin D. (2004a). Therapist alienation: Foreseeing and forestalling third-party dynamics undermining psychotherapy with children of conflicted caregivers. *Professional Psychology: Research and Practice, 35*(4):357–63.

Garber, Benjamin D. (2004b). Parental alienation in light of attachment theory: Consideration of the broader Implications for child development, clinical practice, and forensic process. *Journal of Child Custody, 1*(4):49–76.

Garber, Benjamin D. (2007). Conceptualizing visitation resistance and refusal in the context of parental conflict, separation, divorce. *Family Court Review, 45*(4): 588–99.

Gardner, Richard A. (1976). *Psychotherapy with children of divorce.* New York: Jason Aronson.

Gardner, Richard A. (1979). Death of a parent. In Joseph D. Noshpitz (Ed.), *Basic handbook of child psychiatry,* Vol. 4, pages 270–283. New York: Basic Books.

Gardner, Richard A. (1982). *Family evaluation in child custody litigation.* Cresskill, New Jersey: Creative Therapeutics.

Gardner, Richard A. (1985). Recent trends in divorce and custody litigation. *Academy Forum, 29*(2):3–7.

Gardner, Richard A. (1986). *Child custody litigation: A guide for parents and mental health professionals.* Cresskill, New Jersey: Creative Therapeutics.

Gardner, Richard A. (1987a). *The parental alienation syndrome and the differentiation between fabricated and genuine child sex abuse.* Cresskill, New Jersey: Creative Therapeutics.

Gardner, Richard A. (1987b). Child custody. In Joseph D. Noshpitz (Ed.), *Handbook of child and adolescent psychiatry,* Vol. 5, pages 637–46. New York: Basic Books.

Gardner, Richard A. (1989a). Family evaluation in child custody mediation, arbitration and litigation. *Family & Conciliation Courts Review, 27*(2):93–96.

Gardner, Richard A. (1989b). Differentiating between bona fide and fabricated allegations of sexual abuse of children. *Journal of the American Academy of Matrimonial Lawyers, 5*:1–25.

Gardner, Richard A. (1991a). Legal and psychotherapeutic approaches to the three types of parental alienation syndrome families: When psychiatry and law join forces. *Court Review, 28*(1):14–21.

Gardner, Richard A. (1991b). *Sex abuse hysteria: Salem witch trials revisited.* Cresskill, New Jersey: Creative Therapeutics.

Gardner, Richard A. (1992a). *The parental alienation syndrome: A guide for Mental health and legal professionals.* Cresskill, New Jersey: Creative Therapeutics.

Gardner, Richard A. (1992b). *True and false allegations of child sex abuse.* Cresskill, New Jersey: Creative Therapeutics.

Gardner, Richard A. (1994). The detrimental effects on women of the misguided gender egalitarianism of the child-custody resolution guidelines. *Academy Forum, 38*(1/2):10–13.

Gardner, Richard A. (1998a). Recommendations for dealing with parents who induce a parental alienation syndrome in their children. *Journal of Divorce & Remarriage, 28*(3–4):1–23.

Gardner, Richard A. (1998b). *The parental alienation syndrome: A guide for mental health and legal professionals* (2nd ed.). Cresskill, New Jersey: Creative Therapeutics.

Gardner, Richard A. (1998c). The Burgess decision and the Wallerstein brief. *Journal of the American Academy of Psychiatry and the Law, 26*(3):425–32.

Gardner, Richard A. (1998d). Letter to the Editor. *Child Maltreatment, 3*(4):309–12.

Gardner, Richard A. (1999a). Family therapy of the moderate type of parental alienation syndrome. *American Journal of Family Therapy, 27*(3):195–212.

Gardner, Richard A. (1999b). Guidelines for assessing parental preference in child-custody disputes. *Journal of Divorce & Remarriage, 30*(1):1–9.

Gardner, Richard A. (1999c). Differentiating between parental alienation syndrome and bona fide abuse-neglect. *American Journal of Family Therapy, 27*(2):97–107.

Gardner, Richard A. (2001a). Should courts order PAS children to visit/reside with the alienated parent? A follow-up study. *American Journal of Forensic Psychology, 19*(3):61–106.

Gardner, Richard A. (2001b). *Therapeutic interventions for children with parental alienation syndrome.* Cresskill, New Jersey: Creative Therapeutics.

Gardner, Richard A. (2001c). Parental alienation syndrome (PAS): Sixteen years later. *Academy Forum, 45*(1):10–12.

Gardner, Richard A. (2001d). Rebuttal to Carol S. Bruch's article, "Parental alienation syndrome and parental alienation: Getting it wrong in child custody cases." *www.pas-konferenz.de/e/dok/garnderbruch_e.doc,* accessed July 3, 2009.

Gardner, Richard A. (2002a). Denial of the parental alienation syndrome also harms women. *American Journal of Family Therapy, 30*(3):191–202.

Gardner, Richard A. (2002b). Parental alienation syndrome vs. parental alienation: Which diagnosis should evaluators use in child-custody disputes? *American Journal of Family Therapy, 30*(2):93–115.

Gardner, Richard A. (2002c). The empowerment of children in the development of parental alienation syndrome. *American Journal of Forensic Psychology, 20*(2):5–29.

Gardner, Richard A. (2002d). Misinformation versus facts about the contributions of Richard A. Gardner, M.D. *American Journal of Family Therapy, 30*(5):395–416.

Gardner, Richard A. (2002e). *Das elterliche Entfremdungssyndrom. Anregungen für gerichtliche Sorge- und Umgangsregelungen [The Parental Alienation Syndrome:*

Suggestions for Judicial Custody and Handling Regulations] [German]. Berlin: Verlag für Wissenschaft und Bildung.

Gardner, Richard A. (2003a). Does DSM-IV have equivalents for the parental alienation syndrome (PAS) diagnosis? *American Journal of Family Therapy, 31*(1):1–21.

Gardner, Richard A. (2003b). The judiciary's role in the etiology, symptom development, and treatment of the parental alienation syndrome (PAS). *American Journal of Forensic Psychology, 21*(1):39–64.

Gardner, Richard A. (2003c). The parental alienation syndrome–Past, present and future. In: *Das Parental Alienation Syndrom: Eine interdisziplinäre Herausforderung für scheidungsbegleitende Berufe,* Eds. Wilfrid von Boch-Galhau et al., pages 89–124. Berlin: Verlag für Wissenschaft und Bildung.

Gardner, Richard A. (2004a). Commentary on Kelly and Johnston's "The alienated child: A reformulation of parental alienation syndrome." *Family Court Review, 42*(4):611–21.

Gardner, Richard A. (2004b). The relationship between the parental alienation syndrome (PAS) and the false memory syndrome (FMS). *American Journal of Family Therapy, 32*(2):79–99.

Gardner, Richard A. (2004c). The three levels of parental alienation syndrome alienators: Differential diagnosis and management. *American Journal of Forensic Psychiatry, 25*(3):41–76.

Gardner, Richard A. (2006a). The parental alienation syndrome and the corruptive power of anger. In Richard A. Gardner, S. Richard Sauber, and Demosthenes Lorandos (Eds.), *The international handbook of parental alienation syndrome: Conceptual, clinical and legal consideration,* pages 33–48. Springfield, Illinois: Charles C Thomas.

Gardner, Richard A. (2006b). Future predictions on the fate of PAS children: What hath alienators wrought? In Richard A. Gardner, S. Richard Sauber, and Demosthenes Lorandos (Eds.), *The international handbook of parental alienation syndrome: Conceptual, clinical and legal consideration,* pages 179–94. Springfield, Illinois: Charles C Thomas.

Gardner, Richard A., S. Richard Sauber, and Demosthenes Lorandos (Eds.). (2006). *The international handbook of parental alienation syndrome: Conceptual, clinical and legal considerations.* Springfield, Illinois: Charles C Thomas.

Garrity, Carla B., and Mitchell A. Baris. (1994). *Caught in the middle: Protecting the children of high-conflict divorce.* New York: Lexington Books.

Gaulier, Bernard, Judith Margerum, Jerome A. Price, and James Windell. (2007). *Defusing the high-conflict divorce: A treatment guide for working with angry couples.* Atascadero, California: Impact Publishers.

Gerhardt, Peter, Bernd von Heintschel-Heinegg, and Michael Klein, Eds. (2008). *Handbuch des Fachanwalts Familienrecht [Handbook for Matrimonial Lawyers]* [German]. Munich: Luchterhand-Verlag.

Giorgi, Roberto. (2005). Le possibili insidie delle Child Custody Disputes: Introduzione critica alla sindrome di Alienazione Parentale di Richard A. Gardner [The possible pitfalls of Child Custody Disputes: Critical Introduction to Parental Alienation Syndrome by Richard A. Gardner] [Italian]. *Nuove Tendenze della Psicologia, 3*:53–74.

Glaser, Barney G., and Anselm C. Strauss. (1967). *The discovery of grounded theory: Strategies for qualitative research.* Piscataway, New Jersey: Transaction Publishers.

Golafshani, Nahid. (2003). Understanding reliability and validity in qualitative research. *Qualitative Report, 8*(4):597–607.

Gold-Greenberg, Linda, and Abraham Worenklein. (2001). L'aliénation parentale, un défi légal et clinique pour les psychologues [Parental alienation, a legal and clinical challenge for psychologists] [French]. *Psychologie Québec* (September 2001):26–27.

Goldwater, Anne-France. (1991). Le syndrome d'aliénation parentale [Parental alienation syndrome] [French]. In: *Développements Récents en Droit Familial,* pages 121–45. Cowansville, Québec: Yvon Blais.

Gómez, Paola Andrea Mina. (2008). Síndrome de Alienación Parental (SAP) [Parental alienation syndrome (PAS)] [Spanish]. *Revista de derecho de familia: Doctrina, Jurisprudencia, Legislación, 38*:63–80.

Goncalves, Pedro, and A. Grimaud de Vincenzi. (2003). D'ennemis à Coéquipiers, le Difficile Apprentissage de la Coparentalité après un Divorce Conflictuel [Co-parenting after a conflicted divorce, growing from enemy to ally] [French]. *Thérapie Familiale, 24*(3):239–53.

Gordon, Robert M. (1998). The Medea complex and the parental alienation syndrome: When mothers damage their daughter's ability to love a man. In Gerd H. Fenchel (Ed.), *The mother-daughter relationship echoes through time,* pages 207–25. Northvale, New Jersey: Jason Aronson.

Gordon, Robert M., Ronald Stoffey, and Jennifer Bottinelli. (2008). MMPI-2 findings of primitive defenses in alienating parents. *American Journal of Family Therapy, 36*(3):211–28.

Gottlieb, Daniel S. (2006). Parental alienation syndrome–An Israeli perspective: Reflections and recommendations. In Richard A. Gardner, S. Richard Sauber, and Demosthenes Lorandos (Eds.), *The international handbook of parental alienation syndrome: Conceptual, clinical and legal consideration,* pages 90–107. Springfield, Illinois: Charles C Thomas.

Goudard, Bénédicte. (2008). Syndrome D'Aliénation Parentale [Parental Alienation Syndrome] [French]. Dissertation, Faculty of Medicine, Lyon-Nord, University Claude Bernard.

Gould, Jonathan W. (2006). *Conducting scientifically crafted child custody evaluations* (2nd ed.). Sarasota, Florida: Professional Resource Press/Professional Resource Exchange.

Granados, Francisco. (1987). Lo irracional en el conflicto familiar [The irrational in family conflict] [Spanish]. *Actualidad Civil, 35*(21):2087–95.

Grattagliano, Ignazio, Nunzia Daniela Liantonio, Isabella Berlingerio, and Rosa Taratufolo. (2009). La sindrome di alienazione genitoriale (PAS) raccontata dai disegni dei bambine: Due casi emblematici [The parental alienation syndrome (PAS) told by drawings of children: Two representative cases] [Italian]. *Rivista di Diritto Minorile, 2*(1):89–96.

Green, Arthur H. (1986). True and false allegations of sexual abuse in child custody disputes. *Journal of the American Academy of Child Psychiatry, 25*(4):449.

Groner, Jonathan. (1991). *Hilary's trial: The Elizabeth Morgan case: A child's ordeal in America's legal system.* New York: Simon & Shuster.

Gulotta, Guglielmo. (1998). La sindrome di alienazione genitoriale: Definizione e descrizione [The parental alienation syndrome: Definition and description] [Italian]. *Pianeta Infanzia, 4.*27–36.

Gulotta, Guglielmo, Adele Cavedon, and Moira Liberatore. (2008). *La Sindrome di Alienazione Parentale (PAS): Lavaggio del cervello e programmazione dei figli in danno dell'altro genitore. [The Parental Alienation Syndrome (PAS): Brainwashing and Programming of Children to the Detriment of the Other Parent]* [Italian]. Milan: Giuffrè.

Haas, Trish Oleska (2004). Child custody determinations in Michigan: Not in the best interests of chldren or parents. *University of Detroit Mercy Law Review, 81:*333.

Hamarman, Stephanie, and William Bernet. (2000). Evaluating and reporting emotional abuse in children: Parent-based, action-based focus aids in clinical decision-making1. *Journal of the American Academy of Child and Adolescent Psychiatry, 39*(7):928–30.

Hannuniemi, Anja. (2007). Vanhemmasta vieraannuttaminen–ulka lasten hyvinvoinnille [Alienating a child from one parent–A threat to children's wellbeing] [Finnish]. *Oikeustiede–Jurispredentia,* :1–126.

Hannuniemi, Anja. (2008a). Vieraannuttamisoireyhtymää koskevien väärinkäsitysten oikaiseminen [Straightening the misunderstandings about PAS] [Finnish]. *Lakimies,* (7–8):1249–60.

Hannuniemi, Anja. (2008b). Lapsen tahdonmuodostus ja vieraannuttamisoireyhtymä huolto- ja tapaamisoikeuskäytännössä [The forming of the child's will and the parental alienation syndrome in the legal praxis of custody and visitation rights] [Finnish]. *Defensor Legis,* (6):992–1016.

Harlow, Harry. (1958). The nature of love. *American Psychologist, 13.*673–85.

Hayez, Jean-Yves, and Philippe Kinoo. (2005). Aliénation parentale: Un concepte à haut risque [The parental alienation syndrome: A high risk concept] [French]. *Neuropsychiatrie de l'Enfance et de l'Adolescence, 53*(4):157–65.

Heinze, Michaela C., and Thomas Grisso. (1996). Review of instruments assessing parenting competencies used in child custody evaluations. *Behavioral Sciences and the Law, 14*(3):293–313.

Hellblom Sjögren, Lena. (1997). *Hemligheter och minnen. Att utreda tillförlitlighet i sexualbrottmål [Secrets and Memories: To Investigate Reliability in Sexual Criminal Cases]* [Swedish]. Stockholm: Norstedts Juridik.

Hellblom Sjögren, Lena. (2001). Farlig eller farliggjord mamma? [A dangerous mother or one that has been made dangerous?] [Swedish]. *Läkartidningen, 98:*47.

Hellblom Sjögren, Lena. (2003). Making a parent dangerous–PAS in Sweden and Norway. In: *Das Parental Alienation Syndrom: Eine interdisziplinäre Herausforderung für scheidungsbegleitende Berufe,* Eds. Wilfrid von Boch-Galhau et al., pages 235–48. Berlin: Verlag für Wissenschaft und Bildung.

Hellblom Sjögren, Lena. (2006). PAS in compulsory public custody conflicts. In Richard A. Gardner, S. Richard Sauber, and Demosthenes Lorandos (Eds.), *The international handbook of parental alienation syndrome: Conceptual, clinical and legal consideration,* pages 131–52. Springfield, Illinois: Charles C Thomas.

Hellblom Sjögren, Lena. (2008a). Behöver psykologen bry sig om PAS? [Does the psychologist have to care about PAS?] [Swedish]. *Psykologtidningen,* (8):25–28.

Hellblom Sjögren, Lena. (2008b). Psykiska övergrepp på barn i de allra svåraste vårdnadskonflikterna [Mental abuse of children in the most severe custody conflicts] [Swedish]. *Juridisk Tidskrift, 19*(4):986–94.

Herman, Steve. (2005). Improving decision making in forensic child sexual abuse evaluations. *Law and Human Behavior, 29*(1):87–120.

Herman, Steve. (2009). Forensic child sexual abuse evaluations. In Kathryn Kuehnle and Mary Connell (Eds.), *The evaluation of child sexual abuse allegations: A comprehensive guide to assessment and testimony,* pages 247–266. Hoboken, New Jersey: John Wiley & Sons.

Hetherington, E. Mavis, Martha Cox, and Roger Cox. (1985). Long-term effects of divorce and remarriage on the adjustment of children. *Journal of the American Academy of Child Psychiatry, 24*(5)518–30.

Hetherington, E. Mavis, and M. Stanley-Hagan. (1999). The adjustment of children with divorced parents: A risk and resiliency perspective. *Journal of Child Psychology and Psychiatry and Allied Disciplines, 40*(1):129–40.

Hetherington, E. Mavis, and John Kelly. (2002). *For better or for worse: Divorce reconsidered.* New York: W. W. Norton.

Heyman, Richard E., Amy M. Smith Slep, Steven R. H. Beach, Marianne Z. Wamboldt, Nadine J. Kaslow, and David Reiss. (2009). Relationship problems and the DSM: Needed improvements and suggested solutions 1. *World Psychiatry, 8*(1):7–14.

Hobbs, Tony. (2002a). Parental alienation syndrome and UK family courts (part 1). *Family Law, 32:*182–89.

Hobbs, Tony. (2002b). Parental alienation syndrome and UK family courts (part 2). *Family Law, 32:*381–87.

Hobbs, Tony. (2006a). PAS in the United Kingdom: Problems in recognition and management. In Richard A. Gardner, S. Richard Sauber, and Demosthenes Lorandos (Eds.), *The international handbook of parental alienation syndrome: Conceptual, clinical and legal consideration,* pages 71–89. Springfield, Illinois: Charles C Thomas.

Hobbs, Tony. (2006b). Legal requirements of experts giving evidence to courts in the United Kingdom: PAS and the experts' failure to comply. In Richard A. Gardner, S. Richard Sauber, and Demosthenes Lorandos (Eds.), *The international handbook of parental alienation syndrome: Conceptual, clinical and legal consideration,* pages 439–50. Springfield, Illinois: Charles C Thomas.

Hodges, William F. (1991). *Interventions for children of divorce: Custody, access, and psychotherapy.* New York: John Wiley & Sons.

Holgerson, Astrid, and Lena Hellblom Sjögren (Eds.). (1997). *Seksuelle overgrep mot barn–et kritisk perspektiv [Child Sexual Abuse–A Critical Perspective]* [Norwegian]. Bergen-Sandviken, Norway: Fagbokforlaget.

Hoppe, Carl F. (1997). Perpetually battling parents. In Bonnie S. Mark and James A. Incorvaia (Eds.), *The handbook of infant, child, and adolescent psychotherapy: New direc-*

tions in integrative treatment. New York: Jason Aronson.

Hoult, Jennifer. (2006). The evidentiary admissibility of parental alienation syndrome: science, law and policy. *Children's Legal Rights Journal, 26*(1):1–61.

Hövel, Gabriele ten. (2003). *Liebe Mama, Böser Papa: Eltern-Kind-Entfremdung nach Trennung und Scheidung: Das PAS-Syndrom [Dear Mom, Bad Dad: Parent-Child Alienation after Separation and Divorce: The PAS Syndrome* [German]. Munich: Kösel.

Hudziak, James J., Thomas M. Achenbach, Robert R. Althoff, and Daniel S. Pine. (2007). A dimensional approach to developmental psychopathology. *International Journal of Methods in Psychiatric Research, 16*(S1):S16–S23.

Hysjulien, Chery, Barbara Wood, and G. Andrew Benjamin. (1994). Child custody evaluations: A review of methods used in litigation and alternative dispute resolution. *Family & Conciliation Courts Review, 32*(4):466–89.

Instituto de Investigaciones Jurícas. (2009). Civil Code of the State of Querétaro, Book I, Title Nine, chapter I, Article 396. *www.juridicas.unam.mx,* accessed November 23, 2009.

Isaacs, Marla Beth, Braulio Montlavo, and David Abelsohn. (1986). *The difficult divorce: Therapy for children and families.* New York: Basic Books.

Isman, Danielle. (1996). Gardner's witch-hunt: A discussion of the theory of parental alienation syndrome. *UC Davis Journal of Juvenile Law and Policy, 1*(1):12.

Jacobs, John W. (1988). Euripides' Medea: A psychodynamic model of severe divorce pathology. *American Journal of Psychotherapy, 42*(2):308–19.

Jaffe, Peter G., Dan Ashbourne, and Alfred A. Mamo. (2010). Early identification and prevention of parent-child alienation: A framework for balancing risks and benefits of intervention. *Family Court Review, 48*(1)136–52.

Jaffe, Peter G., Janet R. Johnston, Claire V. Crooks, and Nicholas Bala. (2008). Custody disputes involving allegations of domestic violence: Toward a differential approach to parenting plans. *Family Court Review, 46*(3):500–23.

Jarne Esparcia, Adolpho, and Mila Arch Marin. (2009). DSM, salud mental y síndrome de alienación parental [DSM, mental health, and parental alienation syndrome] [Spanish]. *Papeles del Psicólogo, 30*(1):86–91.

Jeffries, Michael. (2009). *A family's heartbreak: A parent's introduction to parental alienation.* Stamford, Connecticut: A Family's Heartbreak, LLC.

Jelalian, Elissa, and Arthur G. Miller. (1984). The perseverance of beliefs: Conceptual perspectives and research developments. *Journal of Social and Clinical Psychology, 2*:25–56.

Jenkins, Suzanne. (2002). Are children protected in the family court? A perspective from Western Australia. *ANZJFT Australian and New Zealand Journal of Family Therapy, 23*(3):145–52.

Jick, Todd D. (1979). Mixing qualitative and quantitative methods: Triangulaton in action. *Administrative Science Quarterly, 24*(4):602–11.

Johnston, Janet R. (1993). Children of divorce who refuse visitation. In C. Depner and J. H. Bray (Eds.), *Non-residential parenting: New vistas in family living,* pages 109–35. Newbury Park, California: Sage.

Johnston, Janet R. (1994). High-conflict divorce. *Future Child, 4*(1):165–82.

Johnston, Janet R. (2003). Parental alignments and rejection: An empirical study of alienation in children of divorce. *Journal of the American Academy of Psychiatry and the Law, 31*(2):158–70.

Johnston, Janet R. (2005). Children of divorce who reject a parent and refuse visitation: Recent research and social policy implications for the alienated child. *Family Law Quarterly, 38*(4):757–75.

Johnston, Janet R., and Linda E. G. Campbell. (1999). *Impasses of divorce: The dynamics and resolution of family conflict.* New York: Free Press.

Johnston, Janet R., Linda E. G. Campbell, and Sharon S. Mayes. (1985). Latency children in post-separation and divorce disputes. *Journal of the American Academy of Child Psychiatry, 24*(5):563–74.

Johnston, Janet R., and Linda K. Girdner. (2001). Family abductors: Descriptive profiles and preventive interventions. *Juvenile Justice Bulletin, 1*:1–7.

Johnston, Janet R., Roberto Gonzalez, and Linda E. Campbell. (1987). Ongoing postdivorce conflict and child disturbance. *Journal of Abnormal Child Psychology, 15*(4):493–509.

Johnston, Janet R., and Joan B. Kelly. (2004a). Rejoinder to Gardner's "Commentary on Kelly and Johnston's 'The alienated child: A reformulation of parental alienation syndrome.'" *Family Court Review, 42*(4):622–28.

Johnston, Janet R., and Joan B. Kelly. (2004b). Commentary on Walker, Brantley, and Rigsbee's (2004) "A Critical Analysis of Parental Alienation Syndrome and Its Admissibility in the Family Court." *Journal of Child Custody, 1*(4):77–89.

Johnston, Janet R., Marsha Kline, and Jeanne M. Tschann. (1989). Ongoing postdivorce conflict: Effects on children of joint custody and frequent access. *American Journal of Orthopsychiatry, 59*(4):576–92.

Johnston, Janet R., Soyoung Lee, Nancy W. Olesen, and Marjorie G. Walters. (2005). Allegations and substantiations of abuse in custody-disputing families. *Family Court Review, 43*(2):283–94.

Johnston, Janet R., and Vivienne Roseby. (1997). Parental alignments and alienation among children of high-conflict divorce. In: *In the name of the child,* pages 193–220. New York: Simon & Schuster.

Johnston, Janet R., Vivienne Roseby, and Kathryn Kuehnle. (2009). *In the name of the child: A developmental approach to understanding and helping children of conflicted and violent divorce* (2nd ed.). New York: Springer Publishing Company.

Johnston, Janet R., Marjorie G. Walters, and Steven Friedlander. (2001). Therapeutic work with alienated children and their families. *Family Court Review, 39*(3):316–33.

Johnston, Janet R., Marjorie G. Walters, and Nancy W. Olesen. (2005a). Clinical ratings of parenting capacity and Rorschach protocols of custody-disputing parents: An exploratory study. *Journal of Child Custody, 2*:159–78.

Johnston, Janet R., Marjorie G. Walters, and Nancy W. Olesen. (2005b). Is it alienating parenting, role reversal or child abuse? A study of children's rejection of a parent in child custody disputes. *Journal of Emotional Abuse, 5*(4):191–218.

Johnston, Janet R., Marjorie G. Walters, and Nancy W. Olesen. (2005c). The psychological functioning of alienated children in custody disputing families: An exploratory study. *American Journal of Forensic Psychology, 23*(3):39–64.

Jones, Colin P. A. (2007). In the best interests of the court: What American lawyers need to know about child custody and visitation in Japan. *University of Hawaii Asian-Pacific Law & Policy Journal, 8*(2):166–269.

Jopt, Uwe, and Katharina Behrend. (2000a). Das Parental Alienation Syndrome (PAS)–Ein Zwei-Phasen-Modell I [The parental alienation syndrome: A two-stage model I] [German]. *Zentralblatt für Jugendrecht, 87*(6):223–31.

Jopt, Uwe, and Katharina Behrend. (2000b). Das Parental Alienation Syndrome (PAS)–Ein Zwei-Phasen-Modell II [The parental alienation syndrome: A two-stage model II] [German]. *Zentralblatt für Jugendrecht, 87*(7):258–71.

Jopt, Uwe, and Julia Zütphen. (2002). Elterliche PASsivität nach Trennung–Zur Bedeutung des betreuenden Elternteils für die PAS-Genese [Parental PASsiveness after separation–About the significance of the custodial parent for the genesis of PAS] [German]. In: *Qualitätssicherung in der Rechtspsychologie,* Eds. Thomas Fabian et al., pages 183–97. Münster: Lit-Verlag.

Joyal, Renée, Anne Quéniart, and Hubert Van Gijseghem. (2005). Enfants en garde partagée: Quelques questions et réponses [Children in joint residential custody: Some questions and answers] [French]. *Intervention,* (122):51–59.

Kamarudin, Zaleha. (2009). When fathers move out of the home. The Star Online, November 10, 2009. *thestar.com.my,* accessed November 13, 2009.

Katona, Esther Theresia. (2007). Parental Alienation Syndrome–Der Verlust des eigenen Kindes durch Trennung und Scheidung: Eine Studie über den Verlauf des Kontaktabbruchs zum eigenen Kind und der daraus resultierenden Auswirkungen auf betroffene Eltern [Parental Alienation Syndrome–A Study on the Course of Contact Disruption and Resulting Effects on Affected Parents] [German]. Dissertation, Institut für Psychologie der Universität Freiburg, Freiburg, Germany.

Katz, Alayne. (2003). Junk science v. novel scientific evidence: Parental alienation syndrome, getting it wrong in custody cases. *Pace Law Review, 24*(1):239–43.

Kelly, Joan B. (2010). Commentary on "Family Bridges: Using insights from social science to reconnect parents and alienated children." *Family Court Review, 48*(1)81–90.

Kelly, Joan B., and Robert E. Emery. (2003). Children's adjustment following divorce: Risk and resilience perspectives. *Family Relations, 52*:352–62.

Kelly, Joan B., and Janet R. Johnston. (2001). The alienated child: A reformulation of parental alienation syndrome. *Family Court Review, 39*(3):249–66.

Kelly, Joan B., and Michael E. Lamb. (2000). Using child development research to make appropriate custody and access decisions for young children. *Family Court Review, 38*(3):297–311.

Kenan, Joseph, and William Bernet. (2009). Parental alienation. In: *Wiley Encyclopedia of Forensic Science,* Vol. 4, Eds. Allan Jamieson and Andres Moenssens, pages 1981–1984. New York: John Wiley & Sons.

Kendler, Kenneth, David Kupfer, William Narrow, Katharine Phillips, and Jan Fawcett. (2009). Guidelines for making changes in DSM-V, Revised October 21, 2009. *www.psych.org,* accessed November 30, 2009.

Kerr, Michael E., and Murray Bowen. (1988). *Family evaluation.* New York: W. W. Norton.

Kihlbom, Magnus. (1998). Relationen till föräldrarna–grunden för barnets psykiska utveckling [The relation to the parents–The foundation for the child's mental development] [Swedish]. In: *Barnets rätt till båda föräldrarna [The Child's Right to Both Parents]*. Falun, Sweden: Rädda Barnen [Save the Children].

King, Michael. (2002). An autopoietic approach to "Parental Alienation Syndrome." *Journal of Forensic Psychiatry, 13*(3):609–35.

Klass, Joanna L., and Joel V. Klass. (2005). Threatened Mother Syndrome (TMS): a diverging concept of Parental Alienation Syndrome (PAS). *American Journal of Family Law, 18*(4):189–91.

Klenner, Wolfgang. (1995). Rituale der Umgangsvereitelung bei getrennt lebenden oder geschiedenen Eltern [Rituals of contact refusal from parents in separation or divorce] [German]. *Zeitschrift für das gesamte Familienrecht, 42*(24):1529–35.

Klenner, Wolfgang. (2002). Szenarien der Entfremdung im elterlichen Trennungs-prozess: Entwurf eines Handlungskonzepts von Prävention und Intervention [Scenarios of alienation in the parental separation process: Design for concept of action for prevention and intervention] [German]. *Zentralblatt für Jugendrecht, 89*(2):48–57.

Knappert, Christine. (2003). Frühe Interventionsstrategien als Möglichkeiten der Jugendamtsmitarbeiter in der Arbeit mit PAS-Fällen [Possible early intervention strategies implemented by social institutions dealing with PAS cases] [German]. In: *Das Parental Alienation Syndrom: Eine interdisziplinäre Herausforderung für schei-dungsbegleitende Berufe,* Eds. Wilfrid von Boch-Galhau et al., pages 333–41. Berlin: Verlag für Wissenschaft und Bildung.

Kodjoe, Ursula. (2000). Auswirkungen des Vater-Kind-Kontaktverlustes: der "imma-terielle Schaden" aus psychologischer Sicht: Anmerkungen zur Elsholz-Entscheidung des Europäischen Gerichtshofs für Menschenrechte [Consequences of father-child contact disruption: The "immaterial loss" from a psychological view-point. Remarks about the Elsholz decision] [German]. *Der Amtsvormund, 73*(8):641–44.

Kodjoe, Ursula. (2003a). Die Auswirkungen von Entfremdung und Kontaktabbruch auf betroffene Eltern [Consequences of alienation and loss of contact for alienat-ed parents] [German]. In: *Das Parental Alienation Syndrom: Eine interdisziplinäre Herausforderung für scheidungsbegleitende Berufe,* Eds. Wilfrid von Boch-Galhau et al., pages 163–66. Berlin: Verlag für Wissenschaft und Bildung.

Kodjoe, Ursula. (2003b). Vorwort [Preface]. In: *Das Parental Alienation Syndrom: Eine interdisziplinäre Herausforderung für scheidungsbegleitende Berufe,* Eds. Wilfrid von Boch-Galhau et al., pages 11–12. Berlin: Verlag für Wissenschaft und Bildung.

Kodjoe, Ursula, and Peter Koeppel. (1998a). The Parental Alienation Syndrome (PAS) I. *Der Amtsvormund, 71*(1):9–26.

Kodjoe, Ursula, and Peter Koeppel. (1998b). The Parental Alienation Syndrome (PAS) II. *Der Amtsvormund, 71*(2):135–40.

Kodjoe, Ursula, and Peter Koeppel. (1998c). Früherkennung von PAS–Möglichkeiten psychologischer und rechtlicher Interventionen [Early diagnosis of PAS–Possibilities of psychological and juridical interventions] [German]. *Kindschaftsrechtliche Praxis, 1*(5):138–44.

Koeppel, Peter. (2000). Zur Bedeutung der "Elsholz-Entscheidung" für die Fortentwicklung des deutschen Kindschaftsrechts: Anmerkungen zum Minderheitsvotum aus Sicht des Verfahrensbevollmächtigten [On the significance of the "Elsholz decision" for the further development of German custody laws: Remarks on the minority votum from the view point of the authorized legal representative] [German]. *Der Amtsvormund, 73*(8):639–42.

Koeppel, Peter. (2001). PAS und das deutsche Kindschaftsrecht (juristischer Aspekt) [PAS and the German custody laws (legal aspect)] [German]. In: *Eltern sägen ihr Kind entzwei–Trennungserfahrungen und Entfremdung von einem Elternteil [Parents Sawing Their Child Apart: Separation Experiences and Alienation of a Parent* [German], Eds. Siegfried Bäuerle and Helgard Moll-Strobel, pages 65–78. Donauwörth, Germany: Auer Verlag.

Kopetski, Leona. (1998a). Identifying cases of parent alienation syndrome, Part I. *Colorado Lawyer, 27*(2):65–68.

Kopetski, Leona. (1998b). Identifying cases of parent alienation syndrome, Part II. *Colorado Lawyer, 27*(3):61–64.

Kopetski, Leona. (2006). Commentary: Parental alienation syndrome. In Richard A. Gardner, S. Richard Sauber, and Demosthenes Lorandos (Eds.), *The international handbook of parental alienation syndrome: Conceptual, clinical and legal considerations,* pages 378–90. Springfield, Illinois: Charles C Thomas.

Kopetski, Leona, Deirdre Conway Rand, and Randy Rand. (2006). Incidence, gender, and false allegations of child abuse: Data on 84 parental alienation syndrome cases. In Richard A. Gardner, S. Richard Sauber, and Demosthenes Lorandos (Eds.), *The international handbook of parental alienation syndrome: Conceptual, clinical and legal consideration,* pages 65–70. Springfield, Illinois: Charles C Thomas.

Kraemer, Helena Chmura, Art Noda, and Ruth O'Hara. (2004). Categorical versus dimensional approaches to diagnosis: Methodological challenges. *Journal of Psychiatric Research, 38*(1):17–25.

Krause, Martin. (2002). PAS und seine Geschwister–Strukturell-systemische Überlegungen zur Gefährdung des Kindeswohls durch sechs verschiedene Muster pathologischer Trennungsbewältigung [PAS and its sisters–Structural-systemic considerations on the risks for the best interests of the child through six different patterns of pathological adjustment to separation] [German]. *Das Jugendamt, 75*(1):2–6.

Krenicky, Katja. (2003). PAS: Parental Alienation Syndrome–oder die Entfremdung eines Kindes von einem Elternteil nach Trennung oder Scheidung [Parental Alienation Syndrome–or the Alienation of a Child From a Parent After Separation or Divorce] [German]. Dissertation, Pädagogische Hochschule Freiburg, Institut für Psychologie, Freiburg, Germany.

Krivacska, James J. (1989). Review of *The parental alienation syndrome and the differentiation between fabricated and genuine child sex abuse. Issues in Child Abuse Accusations, 1*(1):55–56.

Kuehnle, Kathryn. (1996). *Assessing allegations of child sexual abuse.* Sarasota, Florida: Professional Resource Press.

Kuehnle, Kathryn. (1998a). Child sexual abuse evaluations: The scientist-practitioner model. *Behavioral Sciences and the Law, 16*(1):5–20.

Kuehnle, Kathryn. (1998b). Ethics and the forensic expert: A case study of child custody involving allegations of child sexual abuse. *Ethics & Behavior, 8*(1):1–18.

Kuehnle, Kathryn, and Mary Connell. (2009). *The evaluation of child sexual abuse allegations: A comprehensive guide to assessment and testimony.* Hoboken, New Jersey: John Wiley & Sons.

Kuehnle, Kathryn, Lyn R. Greenberg, and Michael C. Gottlieb. (2004). Incoporating the principles of scientifically based child interviews into family law cases. *Journal of Child Custody, 1*(1):97–114.

Kuehnle, Kathryn, and H. D. Kirkpatrick. (2005). Evaluating allegations of child sexual abuse within complex child custody cases. *Journal of Child Custody, 2*(3):3–39.

Kvilhaug, Sverre. (2005). *Atskillelse barn og foreldre, Hva internasjonal forskning sier om sammenheng mellom atskillelse I barndommen og senere fysiske og psykiske lidelser [Separation of Children and Parents: What International Research Says about the Relationship between Childhood Separation and Later Physical and Mental Disorders]* [Norwegian]. Isdalstö, Norway: Cita Forlag.

Labner, Irene. (2005). Entfremdung im Vater-Kind-Kontakt nach der Scheidung [Alienation in the father-child contact after the divorce] [German]. Dissertation, Universität Innsbruck, Innsbruck, Austria.

Lamontagne, Paule. (1999). Syndrome d'Aliénation Parentale: Contexte et pièges de l'intervention [Parental alienation syndrome: Context and pitfalls regarding intervention] [French] In: *Us et abus de la mise en mots en matière d'abus sexuel [Uses and Abuses of the Discourse Touching upon Sexual Abuse]*, Ed. Hubert Van Gijseghem, pages 177–200. Montreal: Méridien.

Lampel, Anita K. (1986). Post-divorce therapy with high conflict families. *Independent Practitioner, 6*(3):22–26.

Lampel, Anita K. (1996). Children's alignment with parents in highly conflicted custody cases. *Family & Conciliation Courts Review, 34*(2):229–39.

Lampel, Anita K. (1999). Use of the Millon Clinical Multiaxial Inventory-III in evaluating child custody litigants. *American Journal of Forensic Psychology, 17*(4):19–32.

Lampel, Anita K. (2002). Assessing for alienation and access in child custody cases: A response to Lee and Olesen. *Family Court Review, 40*(2):232–35.

Lasbats, Mireille. (2004). Étude du syndrome d'aliénation parentale à partir d'une expertise civile [Study of the parental alienation syndrome from a civil expertise] [French]. *Actualité Juridique Famille,* (11):397–99.

Lee, S. Margaret, and Nancy W. Olesen. (2001). Assessing for alienation in child custody and access evaluations. *Family Court Review, 39*(3):282–98.

Leitner, Werner, and G. Bamberg. (1998). Intervention guided single case help and parental alienation syndrome (PAS): Differential diagnosis and treatment approaches. In Sandra Sebre, Malgozata Rascevska, and Solveiga Miezite (Eds.), *Identity & self esteem: Interactions of students, family, & society,* pages 253–60. Riga, Latvia: SIA.

Leitner, Werner. (2004). Bindungsentwicklung und Bindungsstoerung unter besonderer Beruecksichtigung des "Parental-Alienation-Syndroms" (PAS). [Attachment development and attachment disorder with special regard to the parental alienation syndrome (PAS)] [German]. In: *Bindungsentwicklung und Bindungsstoerung,* Ed. Klaus Udo Ettrich, pages 51–58. Stuttgart: Thieme.

Leitner, Werner, and Annelie Künneth. (2006). Parental alienation syndrome: Theory and practice in Germany. In Richard A. Gardner, S. Richard Sauber, and Demosthenes Lorandos (Eds.), *The international handbook of parental alienation syndrome: Conceptual, clinical and legal consideration,* pages 108–20. Springfield, Illinois: Charles C Thomas.

Leving, Jeffrey M. (2006). The parental alienation syndrome and gender bias in the courts. In Richard A. Gardner, S. Richard Sauber, and Demosthenes Lorandos (Eds.), *The international handbook of parental alienation syndrome: Conceptual, clinical and legal consideration,* pages 391–96. Springfield, Illinois: Charles C Thomas.

Levy, Alan M. (1982). Disorders of visitation in child custody cases. *Journal of Psychiatry and Law, 10*(4):471–89.

Levy, David L. (1992). Review of parental alienation syndrome: A guide for mental health and legal professionals. *American Journal of Family Therapy, 20*(3):276–77.

Levy, David L. (2006). The need for public awareness and policy makers to respond to PAS: A neglected form of child abuse. In Richard A. Gardner, S. Richard Sauber, and Demosthenes Lorandos (Eds.), *The international handbook of parental alienation syndrome: Conceptual, clinical and legal consideration,* pages 153–62. Springfield, Illinois: Charles C Thomas.

Levy, David M. (1943). *Maternal overprotection.* New York: Columbia University Press.

Levy, David M. (1970). The concept of maternal overprotection. In E. James Anthony and Therese Benedek (Eds.), *Parenthood: Its psychology and psychopathology.* Boston: Little, Brown and Company.

Lewis, Ken. (2009). *Child custody evaluations by social workers.* Washington, D.C.: NASW Press.

Loeb, Laurence. (1986). Fathers and sons: Some effects of prolonged custody litigation. *Bulletin of the American Academy of Psychiatry and the Law, 14*(2):177–83.

Lorandos, Demosthenes. (2006a). Parental alienation syndrome in American law. In Richard A. Gardner, S. Richard Sauber, and Demosthenes Lorandos (Eds.), *The international handbook of parental alienation syndrome: Conceptual, clinical and legal consideration,* pages 333–51. Springfield, Illinois: Charles C Thomas.

Lorandos, Demosthenes. (2006b). Parental alienation syndrome: Detractors and the junk science vacuum. In Richard A. Gardner, S. Richard Sauber, and Demosthenes Lorandos (Eds.), *The international handbook of parental alienation syndrome: Conceptual, clinical and legal consideration,* pages 397–418. Springfield, Illinois: Charles C Thomas.

Lord Chancellor's Advisory Board on Family Law. (2002). *Making contact work: A report to the Lord Chancellor on the facilitation of arrangements for contact between children and their non-residential parents and the enforcement of court orders for contact.* London: The Stationery Office.

Lowenstein, Ludwig F. (1998). Parent alienation syndrome: A two-step approach toward a solution. *Contemporary Family Therapy: An International Journal, 20*(4): 505–20.

Lowenstein, Ludwig F. (1999a). Parental alienation and the judiciary. *Medico-legal Journal, 67*(Pt 3):121–23.

Lowenstein, Ludwig F. (1999b). Parental alienation syndrome (PAS). *Justice of the Peace, 163*(4):171–74.

Lowenstein, Ludwig F. (2001). Tackling parental alienation. *Justice of the Peace, 165*(6):102.

Lowenstein, Ludwig F. (2002). Problems suffered by children due to the effects of parental alienation syndrome (PAS). *Justice of the Peace, 166*(24):464–66.

Lowenstein, Ludwig F. (2003). Tackling parental alienation: A summary. *Justice of the Peace, 167*(3):29–30.

Lowenstein, Ludwig F. (2006a). Overturning the programming of a child. *Journal of Parental Alienation, 1*(5):1–12.

Lowenstein, Ludwig F. (2006b). Signs of PAS and how to counteract its effects. *Journal of Parental Alienation, 2*(2):26–30.

Lowenstein, Ludwig F. (2006c). The psychological effects and treatment of parental alienation syndrome. In Richard A. Gardner, S. Richard Sauber, and Demosthenes Lorandos (Eds.), *The international handbook of parental alienation syndrome: Conceptual, clinical and legal consideration,* pages 292–301. Springfield, Illinois: Charles C Thomas.

Lowenstein, Ludwig F. (2007). *Parental alienation: How to understand and address parental alienation resulting from acrimonious divorce or separation.* Lyme Regis, Dorset, UK: Russell House Publishing.

Lowenstein, Ludwig F. (2008). Reducing the hostility. *Justice of the Peace, 172*(20): 322–24.

Lubrano Lavadera, Anna, and Maurizio Marasco. (2005). La sindrome di alienazione genitoriale nelle consulenze tecniche d'ufficio: Uno studio pilota [The parental alienation syndrome and the psychological expert: A pilot study] [Italian]. *Maltrattamento e abuso all'infanzia, 7*(3):63–88.

Luengo Ballester, Domènec, and Arantxa Coca Vila. (2007). *Hijos manipulados tras la separación–Cómo detectar y tratar la alienación parental [Children Manipulated after Separation–How to Detect and Treat Parental Alienation] [Spanish].* Barcelona: Viena Ediciones.

Luengo Ballester, Domènec, and Arantxa Coca Vila. (2009). *El sindrome de alienación parental–80 preguntas y respuestas [The Parental Alienation Syndrome–80 Questions and Answers] [Spanish].* Barcelona: Viena Ediciones.

Luepnitz, Deborah Anna. (1982). *Child custody: A study of families after divorce.* New York: Free Press.

Luiz Silva, Evandro. (2009). *Perícias Psicológicas Nas Varas De Família [Psychological Skills in Family Courts] [Portuguese].* Porto Alegre, Brazil: Editora Equilíbrio.

Luftman, Virginia H., Lane J. Veltkamp, James J. Clark, Sharon Lannacone, and Howard Snooks. (2005). Practice guidelines in child custody evaluations for licensed clinical social workers. *Clinical Social Work Journal, 33*(3):327–57.

Lund, Mary (1995). A therapist's view of parental alienation syndrome. *Family & Conciliation Courts Review, 33*(3):308–16.

Maccoby, Eleanor E., and Robert H. Mnookin. (1992). *Dividing the child: Social and legal dilemmas of custody.* Cambridge, Massachusetts: Harvard University Press.

Maccoby, Eleanor E., Christy M. Buchanan, Robert H. Mnookin, and Sanford M. Dornbusch (1993). Postdivorce roles of mothers and fathers in the lives of their children. *Journal of Family Psychology, 7*(1):24–38.

Machuca, Luisa Pederson. (2005). Parental alienation syndrome: Perceptions of parental behaviors and attitudes in divorced vs. non-divorced families. Dissertation, University of Alaska, Anchorage, Alaska.

Maidment, Susan. (1998). Parental alienation syndrome–A judicial response? *Family Law, 28:*264–66.

Major, Jayne A. (2000). *Breakthrough parenting: Moving your family from struggle to cooperation.* Los Angeles: Breakthrough Parenting Services.

Major, Jayne A. (2006). Helping clients deal with parental alienation syndrome. In Richard A. Gardner, S. Richard Sauber, and Demosthenes Lorandos (Eds.), *The international handbook of parental alienation syndrome: Conceptual, clinical and legal consideration,* pages 276–85. Springfield, Illinois: Charles C Thomas.

Malagoli Togliatti, Marisa, and Marta Franci. (2005). La sindrome di alienazione genitoriale (PAS): Studi e ricerche [The parental alienation syndrome (PAS): Studies and research] [Italian]. *Maltrattamento e abuso all'infanzia, 7*(3):39–63.

Malagoli Togliatti, Marisa, and Anna Lubrano Lavadera. (2005). La sindrome di alienazione genitoriale (PAS): Epigenesi relazionali [The parental alienation syndrome (PAS): Epigenesis of relationships] [Italian]. *Maltrattamento e abuso all'infanzia, 7*(3):7–12.

Malagoli Togliatti, Marisa, Anna Lubrano Lavadera, and Marta Franci. (2005). Les enfants du divorce comme protagonistes actifs de la séparation conjugale [The children of divorce as active protagonists in the parental separation] [French]. *Cahiers critiques de thérapie familiale et de pratiques de réseaux, 34*(1):135–56.

Manonelles, Graciela N. (2005). *Responsabilidad penal del padre obstaculizador, La. Ley 24270. Síndrome de alienación parental (SAP) [Criminal Responsibility of the Obstructing Parent, Law 24270. Parental Alienation Syndrome (PAS)]* [Spanish]. Buenos Aires: Ad-Hoc.

Mart, Eric G. (2007). *Issue focused forensic child custody assessment.* Sarasota, Florida: Professional Resources Press.

Martinson, Donna J. (2010). One case–one specialized judge: Why courts have an obligation to manage alienation and other high-conflict cases. *Family Court Review, 48*(1)180–89.

Mazzoni, Giuiana, and Amina Memon. (2003). Imagination can create false autobiographical memories. *Psychological Science, 14*(2):186–88.

Meadow, Roy. (1993). False allegations of abuse and Munchausen syndrome by proxy. *Archives of Disease in Childhood, 68*(4):444.

Meister, Ron. (2003). Review of *Therapeutic Interventions for Children with Parental Alienation Syndrome. American Journal of Family Therapy, 31*(4):321–24.

Mendelson, Robert. (1998). *A family divided: A divorced father's struggle with the child custody industry.* Amherst, New York: Prometheus Books.

Mercer, Diana, and Marsha Kline Pruett. (2001). *Your divorce advisor.* New York: Simon & Schuster.

Meyer, Catherine L., and Sally Quinn. (1999). *They are my children, too: A mother's struggle for her sons.* New York: PublicAffairs.

Minunchin, Salvador. (1974). *Families and family therapy.* Cambridge, Massachusetts: Harvard University Press.

Mitcham-Smith, Michelle, and Wilma J. Henry. (2007). High-conflict divorce solutions: Parenting coordination as an innovative co-parenting intervention. *Family Journal, 15*(4):368–73.

Mitchell, John. (2002). Parental alienation and the courts. *Medico-legal Journal, 70*(Pt 4):194–95.

Moné, Jennifer Gerber, and Zeynep Biringen. (2006). Perceived parent-child alienation: Empirical assessment of parent-child relationships within divorced and intact families. *Journal of Divorce & Remarriage, 45*(3–4):131–56.

Moné, Jennifer Gerber. (2008). Family Members' Narratives on Divorce and Interparental Conflict. Dissertation, Colorado State University, Fort Collins, Colorado.

Morrison, Stephen L. (2006). Parental Alienation Syndrome: An Inter-Rater Reliability Study. Alienating Behaviors–Related Justice System Issues. Dissertation, University of Southern Mississippi, Hattiesburg, Mississippi.

Moskopp, Stefanie. (2006). The Parental Alienation Syndrome (PAS)–Das Elterliche Entfremdungssyndrom–Möglichkeiten der Intervention und kritische Reflexion [The Parental Alienation Syndrome (PAS)–Possibilities for Intervention and Critical Reflection] [German]. Dissertation, Fachhochschule Koblenz, Koblenz, Germany.

Moss, Debra Cassens. (1988). Teaching kids to hate. *ABA Journal, 74*:19–20.

Murray, Kathleen. (1999). When children refuse to visit parents: Is prison an appropriate remedy? *Family Court Review, 37*(1):83–98.

Namyslowska, Irena, Janusz Heitzman, and Anna Siewierska. (2009). Zespół Gardnera–zespół oddzielenia od drugoplanowego opiekuna (PAS). Rozpoznanie czy rzeczywistosc rodzinna? [Gardner Syndrome–Parent Alienation Syndrome (PAS). Diagnosis or family reality?] [Polish]. *Psychiatria Polska,* (1):5–17.

Napp-Peters, Anneke. (1995). *Familien nach der Scheidung [Families after divorce]* [German]. Munich, Germany: Verlag Antje Kunstmann.

Napp-Peters, Anneke. (2005). Mehrelternfamilien als "Normal"-Familien–Ausgrenzung und Eltern-Kind-Entfremdung nach Trennung und Scheidung [Multi-parent families as "normal" families–Segregation and parent-child-alienation after separation and divorce] [German]. *Praxis der Kinderpsychologie und Kinderpsychiatrie, 54*(10):792–801.

National Council of Juvenile and Family Court Judges. (2006). *Navigating custody & visitation evaluations in cases with domestic violence: A judge's guide.* Reno, Nevada: National Council of Juvenile and Family Court Judges.

National Interdisciplinary Colloquium on Child Custody Law. (1998). *Legal and mental health perspectives on child custody law: A deskbook for judges.* Eagan, Minnesota: West Group.

Neustein, Amy, and Michael Lesher. (2009). Evaluating PAS: A critique of Elizabeth Ellis's "A stepwise approach to evaluating children for PAS." *Journal of Child*

Custody, 6:322–25.

Ney, Tara. (1995). *True and false allegations of child sexual abuse: Assessment and case management.* New York: Brunner/Mazel Publisher.

Nicholas, Larry. (1997). Does parental alienation syndrome exist? Preliminary empirical study of the phenomenon in custody and visitation disputes. *Proceedings of Thirteenth Annual Symposium of the American College of Forensic Psychology,* Vancouver, British Columbia.

Nicholson, E. Bruce, and Josephine Bulkley, Eds. (1988). *Sexual abuse allegations in custody and visitation cases.* Washington, D.C.: American Bar Association.

Niggemyer, Kathleen. (1998). Parental alienation is open heart surgery: It needs more than a band-aid to fix it. *California Western Law Review, 34*:567–89.

Novák, Tomás. (2005). Syndrom zavržení se nemusí týkat jen vztahu rodiče a dítěte [PAS does not have to involve a parent and a child only] [Czech]. *Právo a rodina,* (11):1.

Novák, Tomás. (2008). Syndrom zavrženého rodiče [Parental alienation syndrome] [Czech]. In: *Vztah otce u syna [Between Father and Son].* Prague: Grada.

Novick, Mark R. (2003). Review of *Therapeutic Interventions for Children with Parental Alienation Syndrome. Journal of the American Academy of Psychoanalysis & Dynamic Psychiatry, 31*(2):418–21.

Nurcombe, Barry, and David F. Partlett. (1994). *Child mental health and the law.* New York: Free Press.

Öberg, Bente, and Gunnar Öberg. (1992). *Pappa, se mig! Om förnekade barn och maktlösa fäder [Father, See Me! About Rejected Children and Powerless Fathers]* [Swedish]. Stockholm: Förlagshuset Gothia.

O'Leary, K. Daniel, and Kirstin C. Moerk. (1999). Divorce, children and the courts: Evaluating the use of the Parent Alienation Syndrome in custody disputes. *Expert Evidence, 7*(2):127–46.

Odinetz, Olga. (2009). L'aliénation parentale, une source de souffrance pour l'enfant. [Parental alienation, a source of suffering for the child] [French]. *Métiers de la petite enfance, 15*(150):8–10 (May 2009).

Odyniec, Hannah. (2005). De l'enfant-otage à l'enfant-soldat: Chroniques de guerres familiales [From child-hostage to child-soldier: Chronical of family wars] [French]. *Divorce et Séparation,* (3):128–37.

Olness, Karen, and Daniel P. Kohen. (1996). *Hypnosis and hypnotherapy with children* (3rd ed.). New York: Guilford Press.

Owusu-Bempah, Kwame. (2007). *Children and separation: Socio-genealogical connectedness perspective.* New York: Routledge/Taylor & Francis Group.

Palmer, Nancy R. (1988). Legal recognition of the parental alienation syndrome. *American Journal of Family Therapy, 16*(4):361–63.

Palmer, Sally E. (2002). Custody and access issues with children whose parents are separated or divorced. *Canadian Journal of Community Mental Health* (4 Suppl):25–38.

Pannier, Jean. (2007). Autorité parentale–Droit de visite et d'hébergement–Aliénation parentale [Parental Authority–Rights of access and accommodation–Parental Alienation] [French]. *La Revue d'Action Juridique et Sociale,* (270):58–62.

Parrini, Antonella. (2008). *Separazioni distruttive tra conflittualità e alienazione. Aspetti psicologici e giuridici [Destructive Separation in the Midst of Conflicts and Alienation. Psychological and Legal Aspects]* [Italian]. Chieti, Italy: Psiconline.

Pavlát, Josef. (2005). Deti v rozvodových sporech: Severoamerické studie (1980–2001) [Children in divorce conflicts: American studies (1980–2001)] [Czech]. *Ceskoslovenska Psychologie, 49*(5):422–31.

Pavlát, Josef, and Marak Šusta. (2008). Deti v rodicovských soudních sporech [Children in parental litigation] [Czech]. *Ceskoslovenska Psychologie, 52*(5):458–67.

Pearl, Peggy S. (1994). Emotional abuse. In James A. Monteleone and Armand E. Brodeur (Eds.), *Child maltreatment: A clinical guide and reference,* pages 259–82. St. Louis: G. W. Medical Publishing.

Pedrosa, Delia Susana, and José María Bouza. (2008). *(SAP) Síndrome de Alienación Parental. Proceso de obstrucción del vínculo entre los hijos y uno de sus progenitores [.(PAS) Parental Alienation Syndrome. Process of Obstructing the Bond between the Child and Parent]* [Spanish]. Buenos Aires: García Alonso.

Perissini da Silva, Denise Maria. (2007). *Psicologia Juridica no Processo Civil Brasileiro [Forensic Psychology in the Context of Brazilian Law]* [Portuguese], 2nd ed. São Paulo, Brazil: Casa do Psicólogo.

Peterson, James L., and Nicholas Zill. (1986). Marital disruption, parent-child relationships, and behavior problems in children. *Journal of Marriage and the Family, 48*(2):295–307.

Pett, Marjorie A., Bruce E. Wampold, Charles W. Turner, and Beth Vaughan-Cole. (1999). Paths of influence of divorce on preschool children's psychosocial adjustment. *Journal of Family Psychology, 13*(2):145–64.

Pickett, Cynthia L., and Marilynn B. Brewer. (2005). The role of exclusion in maintaining ingroup inclusion. In Dominic Abrams, Michael A. Hogg, and Jose M. Marques (Eds.), *The social psychology of inclusion and exclusion,* pages 89–112. New York: Psychology Press.

Pollack, Daniel, and Susan Mason. (2004). In the best interest of the child. *Family Court Review, 42*(01):74–84.

Poole, Debra A., and Michael E. Lamb. (1998). *Investigative interviews of children: A guide for helping professionals.* Washington, D. C.: American Psychological Association.

Pressmann, Robert M. (2007). Review of *The international handbook of parental alienation syndrome. American Journal of Family Therapy, 35*(3):284–85.

Price, Joseph L., and Kerry S. Pioske. (1994). Parental alienation syndrome. A developmental analysis of a vulnerable population. *Journal of Psychosocial Nursing and Mental Health Services, 32*(11):9–12.

Primo, Franceso. (2008). Sindrome D'Alienazione Genitoriale (PAS) e Sospetto Abuso Sessuale Infantile [Parental Alienation Syndrome (PAS) and Suspicion of Child Sexual Abuse] [Italian]. Dissertation, Università degli Studi di Bari, Bari, Italy.

Pruett, Kyle D., and Marsha Kline Pruett, Eds. (2009). *Child and adolescent psychiatric clinics of North America: Child custody.* New York: W. B. Saunders.

Pruett, Marsha Kline, and D. Mercer. (2002). *Your divorce advisor: A lawyer and a psy-*

chologist guide you through the legal and emotional landscape of divorce. New York: Simon and Schuster.

Racusin, Robert, Stuart A. Copans, and Peter Mills. (1994). Characteristics of families of children who refuse post-divorce visits. *Journal of Clinical Psychology, 50:*792–801.

Ragland, Erika Rivera, and Hope Fields. (2003). Parental alienation syndrome: What professionals need to know, Part 1 of 2. *NCPCA Update Newsletter, 16*(6).

Ramírez González, Marta. (2004). Psicología y derecho de familia. Trastorno mental y alternativa de custodia. El síndrome de alienación parental [Psychology and family law. Mental disorder and alternative care. Parental Alienation Syndrome] [Spanish]. *Psicopatología Clínica Legal y Forense, 4*(1–3):147–54.

Rand, Deirdre Conway. (1997a). The spectrum of parental alienation syndrome (Part I). *American Journal of Forensic Psychology, 15*(3):23–52.

Rand, Deirdre Conway. (1997b). The spectrum of parental alienation syndrome (Part II). *American Journal of Forensic Psychology, 15*(4):39–92.

Rand, Deirdre Conway. (in press) The spectrum of parental alienation syndrome (Part IV): Critics of parental alienation syndrome and the politics of science (Part I). *American Journal of Family Therapy.*

Rand, Deirdre Conway, and Randy Rand. (2006). Factors affecting reconciliation between the child and target parent. In Richard A. Gardner, S. Richard Sauber, and Demosthenes Lorandos (Eds.), *The international handbook of parental alienation syndrome: Conceptual, clinical and legal considerations,* pages 163–76. Springfield, Illinois: Charles C Thomas.

Rand, Deirdre Conway, Randy Rand, and Leona Kopetski. (2005). The spectrum of parental alienation syndrome (Part III): The Kopetski follow-up study. *American Journal of Forensic Psychology, 23*(1):15–43.

Raso, Cynthia. (2004). "If the Bread Goes Stale, It's My Dad's Fault": The Parental Alienation Syndrome. Dissertation, Concordia University, Montreal, Quebec.

Reay, Kathleen M. (2007). Psychological distress among adult children of divorce who perceive experiencing parental alienation syndrome in earlier years. Dissertation, Capella University, Minneapolis, Minnesota.

Reich, Wilhelm. (1945, 2006). *Charakteranalyse [Character Analysis]* [German] (8th ed.). Cologne, Germany: Kiepenheuer & Witsch.

Reich, Wilhelm. (1949). *Character analysis* (3rd ed.). New York: Orgone Institute Press.

Reischer, H. (1999). Review of *The parental alienation syndrome: A guide for mental health and legal professionals. Journal of the American Academy of Child and Adolescent Psychiatry, 27*(3):504–06.

Reppucci, N. Dickon. (1984). The wisdom of Solomon: Issues in child custody determinations. In N. Dickon Reppucci et al. (Eds.), *Children, mental health, and the law.* Thousand Oaks, California: Sage Publications.

Rexilius, Günter. (1999). Kindeswohl und PAS. Zur aktuellen Diskussion des Parental Alienation Syndrome [The best interests of the child and PAS. The ongoing discussion of parental alienation syndrome] [German]. *Kindschaftsrechtliche Praxis, 2:*149–59.

Richardson, Pamela. (2006). *A kidnapped mind: A mother's heartbreaking memoir of parental alienation.* Toronto: Dundurm.

Rohrbaugh, Joanna Bunker. (2008). *A comprehensive guide to child custody evaluations: Mental health and legal perspectives.* New York: Springer Science + Business Media.

Roseby, Vivienne, and Janet R. Johnston. (1995). Clinical interventions with latency-age children of high conflict and violence. *American Journal of Orthopsychiatry, 65*(1):48–59.

Roseby, Vivienne, and Janet R. Johnston. (1998). Children of Armageddon. Common developmental threats in high-conflict divorcing families. *Child and Adolescent Psychiatric Clinics of North America, 7*(2):295–309.

Ross, Lee, Mark R. Lepper, and Michael Hubbard. (1975). Perseverance in self-perception and social perception: Biased attribution processes in the debriefing paradigm. *Journal of Personality and Social Psychology, 32*(5):880–92.

Rueda, Carlos A. (2003). Parental Alienation Syndrome: An Inter-Rater Reliability Study. Dissertation, Walden University.

Rueda, Carlos A. (2004). An inter-rater reliability study of parental alienation syndrome. *American Journal of Family Therapy, 32*(5):391–403.

Salluzzo, Mario Andrea. (2004). Psicopatologia nella separazione, divorzio e affidamento [Psychopathology in separation, divorce and custody] [Italian]. *Attualità in Psicologia, 19*(3/4):221–35.

Salluzzo, Mario Andrea. (2006). La sindrome di alienazione genitoriale (PAS): psicopatologia e abuso dell'affidamento nelle separazione. Interventi di confine tra psicologia e giustizia [The parental alienation syndrome (PAS): Psychopathology and abuse of custody in separation. Borderline interventions between psychology and justice.] [Italian]. *Rivista Scientifica di Psicologia, 8*(January):6–18.

Sauber, S. Richard. (2006). PAS as a family tragedy: Roles of family members, professionals, and the justice system. In Richard A. Gardner, S. Richard Sauber, and Demosthenes Lorandos (Eds.), *The international handbook of parental alienation syndrome: Conceptual, clinical and legal consideration,* pages 12–32. Springfield, Illinois: Charles C Thomas.

Sauber, S. Richard. (2007). Review of *Adult Children of Parental Alienation Syndrome. American Journal of Family Therapy, 35*(4):385–86.

Schacht, Thomas E. (1999). Prevention strategies to protect professionals and families involved in high-conflict divorce. *University of Arkansas at Little Rock Law Review, 22*:565–81.

Schade, Burkhard. (2002). Umgangsregelung gegen den "Kindeswillen"? [Visitation order against the "child's will"] [German]. In: *Qualitätssicherung in der Rechtspsychologie,* Eds. Thomas Fabian et al., pages 213–22. Münster: Lit-Verlag.

Schauss, Scott L., Phillip N. Chase, and Robert Hawkins. (1997). Environment-behavior relations, behavior therapy, and the process of persuasion and attitude change. *Journal of Behavior Therapy and Experimental Psychiatry, 28*(1):31–40.

Schepard, Andrew. (2001). Editorial notes. *Family Court Review, 39*(3):243–45.

Schetky, Diane H. and Elissa P. Benedek, Eds. (2001). *Principles and practice of child and adolescent forensic psychiatry.* Washington, D.C.: American Psychiatric Publishing.

Schmidt, Elisabeth and Allard Mees, Eds. (2006). *Vergiss, dass es Dein Vater ist! Ehemals entfremdete Kinder im Gespräch [Remember that it is your father. Formerly Alienated Children in Conversation]* [German]. Norderstedt, Germany: Books on Demand.

Schreier, Herbert A. (1996). Repeated false allegations of sexual abuse presenting to sheriffs: When is it Munchausen by proxy? *Child Abuse & Neglect, 20*(10):985–91.

Schultz, Glen C. (2007). *Unlawful flight: A parental kidnapping.* New York: Wind Blown Books.

Schutz, Benjamin M., Ellen B. Dixon, Joanne C. Lindberger, and Neil J. Ruther. (1989). *Solomon's sword: A practical guide to conducting child custody evaluations.* San Francisco: Jossey-Bass Publishers.

Schütz, Harald. (2003). Familie und Verantwortung–Nachdenkliche Anmerkungen eines deutschen Familienrichters [Family and responsibility–Comments for reflection of a German family judge] [German]. In: *Das Parental Alienation Syndrom: Eine interdisziplinäre Herausforderung für scheidungsbegleitende Berufe,* Eds. Wilfrid von Boch-Galhau et al., pages 85–88. Berlin: Verlag für Wissenschaft und Bildung.

Segura, C., M. J. Gil, and M. A. Sepúlveda. (2006). El sindrome de alienación parental: una forma de maltrato infantil [The parental alienation syndrome: A form of child abuse] [Spanish]. *Cuadernos de Medicina Forense,* (43–44):117–28.

Sheffner, David J., and John M. Suarez. (1975). The postdivorce clinic. *American Journal of Psychiatry, 132*(4):442–444.

Sherif, Muzafer, O. J. Harvey, B. Jack White, William R. Hood, and Carolyn W. Sherif. (1988). *The Robbers cave experiment.* Middletown, Connecticut: Wesleyan University Press.

Shopper, Moisy. (2005). Parental alienation: The creation of a false reality. In Linda unsberg and Paul Hymowitz (Eds.), *A handbook of divorce and custody: Forensic, developmental, and clinical perspective,* pages 109–25. Hillsdale, New Jersey: Analytic Press.

Siegel, Jeffrey C. (1996). Traditional MMPI-2 validity indicators and initial presentation in custody evaluations. *American Journal of Forensic Psychology, 14*(3):55–64.

Siegel, Jeffrey C., and Joseph S. Langford. (1998). MMPI-2 validity scales and suspected parental alienation syndrome. *American Journal of Forensic Psychology, 16*(4):5–14.

Simons, Virginia, Linda S. Grossman, and Barbara J. Weiner. (1990). A study of families in high-conflict custody disputes: Effects of psychiatric evaluation. *Bulletin of the American Academy of Psychiatry and the Law, 18*(1):85–97.

Sinha, Awadhesh K., Akhileshwar P. Singh, and Asha Kumari (1988). Parent evaluation as a function of sex and alienation. *Indian Journal of Current Psychological Research, 3*(1):29–33.

Skoler, Glen. (1998). A psychological critique of international child custody and abduction law. *Family Law Quarterly, 32*(3):557–602.

Sobal, Barbara Bevando. (2006). Parental alienation syndrome and international child abduction: A multigenerational syndrome. In Richard A. Gardner, S. Richard Sauber, and Demosthenes Lorandos (Eds.), *The international handbook of parental alienation syndrome: Conceptual, clinical and legal consideration,* pages 433–38.

Springfield, Illinois: Charles C Thomas.

Sobal, Barbara Bevando, and William M. Hilton. (2002). Article 13(b) of The Hague Convention Treaty: Does it create a loophole for parental alienation syndrome ('PAS')–An insidious abduction? *International Lawyer, 35*(3):997–1025.

Spangenberg, Brigitte, and Ernst Spangenberg. (2002). Induzierte Umgangsverweigerung (PAS) und Richterliche Kreativität [Induced visitation refusal (PAS) and creativity of judges] [German]. *Familie, Partnerschaft und Recht, 8*(6):256–57.

Spruijt, Ed, Martijn de Goede, and Inge Vandervalk. (2004). Frequency of contact with non-resident fathers and adolescent well-being: A longitudinal analysis. *Journal of Divorce & Remarriage, 40*(3–4):77–90.

Spruijt, Ed, Bianca Eikelenboom, Janneke Harmeling, Robin Stokkers, and Helga Kormos. (2005). Parental Alienation Syndrome (PAS) in the Netherlands. *American Journal of Family Therapy, 33*(4):303–17.

Stahl, Philip M. (1994). *Conducting child custody evaluations.* Thousand Oaks, California: Sage.

Stahl, Philip M. (1999a). *Complex issues in child custody evaluations.* Thousand Oaks, California: Sage.

Stahl, Philip M. (1999b). Personality traits of parents and developmental needs of children in high-conflict families. *Academy of Certified Family Law Specialists Newsletter,* Winter 1999 (3):8–16.

Stahl, Philip M. (1999c). Alienation and alignment of children. *California Psychologist, 32*(3):23–29.

Stahl, Philip M. (2003). Understanding and evaluating alienation in high-conflict custody cases. *Wisconsin Journal of Family Law, 24*(1):20–26.

Stahl, Philip M. (2007). *Parenting after divorce: Resolving conflicts and meeting your children's needs* (2nd ed.). Atascadero, California: Impact Publishers.

Stamps, Leighton E., Seth Kunen, and Anita Rock-Faucheux. (1998). Judges' beliefs dealing with child custody decisions. *Journal of Divorce & Remarriage, 28*(1):3–16.

Steinberger, Chaim. (2006a). Father? What father? Parental alienation and its effect on children. Part I. *Family Law Review, 38*(1):10–24.

Steinberger, Chaim. (2006b). Father? What father? Parental alienation and its effect on children. Part II. *Family Law Review, 38*(2):9–14.

Stephens, Richard. (2009a). The Long History of PAS. *http://glennsacks.com/blog/?= 3825,* accessed June 11, 2009.

Stephens, Richard. (2009b). *A historical perspective on parental alienation and child custody disputes: 1760–Present.* Unpublished manuscript.

Stett, Dietmar. (2009). Auswirkung des elterlichen Konfliktniveaus auf betroffene Scheidungskinder: Empirische Untersuchung anhand einer Scheidungskindergruppe [Effects of parental conflict level on affected children of divorce: Empirical research based on a group for children whose parents are divorced] [German]. Dissertation, Universität Augsburg, Augsburg, Germany.

Stoltz, Jo-Anne M., and Tara Key. (2002). Resistance to visitation: Rethinking parental and child alienation. *Family Court Review, 40*(2):220–31.

Stone, Lawrence. (1993). *Broken lives: Separation and divorce in England, 1660–1857.*

Oxford: Oxford University Press.

Stoner-Moskowitz, Jodi. (1998). The Effect of Parental Alienation Syndrome and Interparental Conflict on the Self-Concept of Children of Divorce. Dissertation, Miami Institute of Psychology of the Caribbean Center for Advanced Studies.

Strauss, Anselm C., Anselm L. Strauss, and Juliet Corbin. (2007). *Basics of qualitative research: Techniques and procedures for developing grounded theory* (3rd ed.). Thousand Oaks, Calif.: Sage.

Stuart-Mills-Hoch, Pamela, and Robert Hoch. (2003). Successful reintegration of severely alienated children and their parents. In: *Das Parental Alienation Syndrom: Eine interdisziplinäre Herausforderung für scheidungsbegleitende Berufe,* Eds. Wilfrid von Boch-Galhau et al., pages 353–65. Berlin: Verlag für Wissenschaft und Bidung.

Sullivan, Matthew, and Joan B. Kelly. (2001). Legal and psychological management of cases with an alienated child. *Family Court Review, 39*(3):299–315.

Sullivan, Matthew, Peggy A. Ward, and Robin M. Deutsch. (2010). Overcoming Barriers Family Camp: A program for high-conflict divorced families where a child is resisting contact with a parent. *Family Court Review, 48*(1)116–35.

Summers, Collette C., and David M. Summers. (2006). Parentectomy in the cross-fire. *American Journal of Family Therapy, 34*(3):243–61.

Summers, David M., and Collete C. Summers. (2006). Unadulterated arrogance: Autopsy of the narcissistic parental alienator. American *Journal of Family Therapy, 34*(5):399–428.

Sutherland, Patricia C. (2002). *Perilous journey: A mother's international quest to rescue her children–A true story.* Far Hills, New Jersey: New Horizon Press.

Szabo, Christopher P. (2002). Parental alienation syndrome. *South African Psychiatry Review, 5*(3):1.

Svarc, Jirí, and Eduard Bakalář. (2004). Syndrom zavrzeného rodice. Príciny, diagnostika, terapie [Parental alienation syndrome: Etiology, diagnostics, therapy] [Czech]. *Prakticky lékar, 84*(1):40–45.

Tejedor Huerta, Asunción. (2006). Reflexiones sobre el Síndrome de Alienación Parental [Thoughts on the parental alienation syndrome] [Spanish]. In: *Nuevos Caminos y Conceptos en la Psicología Jurídica [New Paths in Psychology and Legal Concepts],* Eds. Thomas Fabian, Claudia Böhm, and Juan Romero. Berlin: Lit Verlag.

Tejedor Huerta, Asunción. (2007a). *El Síndrome de Alienación Parental una forma de maltrato [Parental Alienation Syndrome is a Form of Abuse]* [Spanish]. Madrid: EOS.

Tejedor Huerta, Asunción. (2007b). Intervención ante el Síndrome de Alienación Parental [Response to the parental alienation syndrome] [Spanish]. *Anuario de psicología jurídica,* (17):79–89.

Tejedor Huerta, Asunción. (2008). SAP y Maltrato [PAS, a Form of Abuse] [Spanish]. In: *Psicologia Juridica. Familia y Victimologia,* Eds. F. J. Rodríguez et al. Oviedo, Spain: Ediciones de la Universidad de Oviedo.

Tejedor Huerta, Asunción. (2009). Pautas de Intervención ante casos de SAP en la familia [Intervention in cases of Parental Alienation Syndrome] [Spanish]. In: *Más Cerca del Hogar" [Closer to Home],* Ed. Javier Urra Portillo. Madrid: Editorial LID.

Texmo, Ole. (2007). *Et langt og vanskelig ord: Om metodisk påvisning av olike typer av foreldrefiendtliggjöring med referanse til Bone & Walsh (1999) kriterier for identifisering av PAS (Parental Alienation Syndrome) [A Long and Difficult Word: The Methodical Detection of Different Types of Parental Alienation with Reference to the Bone & Walsh (1999) Criteria for the Identification of PAS (Parental Alienation Syndrome)]* [Norwegian]. *www.krisesenter.org/oletexmo,* accessed January 25, 2010.

Thuen, Frode. (2004). *Livet Som Deltidsforeldre [Life as a Part Time Parent] [Norwegian].* Bergen, Norway: Fagbokforlaget.

Torgersen, Terje. (1995a). Vitenskap og synsing [Science and believing] [Norwegian]. *Aftenposten,* February 24, 1995. Oslo, Norway.

Torgersen, Terje. (1995b). Foreldrehat-syndromet [The parental hate syndrome] [Norwegian]. *Aftenposten,* March 10, 1995. Oslo, Norway.

Torgersen, Terje. (2008a). Konflikt som maktmedel [Conflict as a power tool] [Norwegian]. *Dagsavisen,* March 7, 2008. Oslo, Norway.

Torgersen, Terje. (2008b). Samvaersrett og avmakt [Visitiation rights and powerlessness] [Norwegian]. *Dagsavisen,* August 6, 2008. Oslo, Norway.

Traube, Raymond B. (2006). Séparations conflictuelles en pédopsychiatrie legale [Conflicting separations in forensic child psychiatry] [French]. *Schweizer Archiv fur Neurologie und Psychiatrie, 157*(6):270–77.

Trémintin, Jacques. (2005). Quand l'enfant se retrouve piégé–L'aliénation parentale [When the child finds himself/herself trapped–Parental alienation] [French]. *Lien Social,* (739):4–14.

Trnka, Vojtěch. (1967). Vliv popouzení proti některému z rodičů na adaptovanost dětí z rozvedených manzelství [The effect of inciting children against the other parent on the adaptability of children from divorced families] [Czech]. *Ceská Pediatrie, 22*(6):468–81.

Trnka, Vojtěch. (1974). *Dětí a Rozvody [Children and Divorce]* [Czech]. Prague, Czech Republic: Avicenum.

Tschann, Jeanne M., Janet R. Johnston, Marsha Kline, and Judith S. Wallerstein. (1990). Conflict, loss, change and parent-child relationships: Predicting children's adjustment during divorce. *Journal of Divorce, 13*(4):1–22.

Tschudi-Winkler, Gertrud. (2006). Eltern-Kind-Entfremdung bei geschiedenen Eltern: Parental Alienation Syndrome (PAS). Syndrom-Enstehung und Auswirkungen auf das Kind sowie Interventionsmöglichkeiten [Parent-Child Alienation in Case of Divorced Parents: Parental Alienation Syndrome (PAS). Syndrome Development and Effects on the Child as well as Possibilities for Intervention] [German]. Dissertation, Fachhochschule Zürich, Zürich.

Turkat, Ira Daniel. (1994). Child visitation interference in divorce. *Clinical Psychology Review, 14*(8):737–42.

Turkat, Ira Daniel. (1995). Divorce related malicious mother syndrome. *Journal of Family Violence, 10*(3):253–64.

Turkat, Ira Daniel. (1997). Management of visitation interference. *Judge's Journal, 36*(2):17–47.

Turkat, Ira Daniel. (2000). Custody battle burnout. *American Journal of Family Therapy, 28*(3):201–15.

Turkat, Ira Daniel. (2002). Parental alienation syndrome: A review of critical issues.

Journal of the American Academy of Matrimonial Lawyers, 18:131–76.

Turkat, Ira Daniel. (2005). False allegations of parental alienation. *American Journal of Family Law, 19*:1–15.

United Nations Children's Fund (UNICEF). (2009). *The state of the world's children*, Special Edition. New York: United Nations Children's Fund.

United States Census Bureau. (2009). Living arrangements of children under 18 years and marital status of parents: 2008. *www.census.gov/population/www/socdemo/hh-fam/cps2008.html*, accessed February 1, 2010.

Urra, Javier .(2009). *Más cerca del hogar [Closer to Home]* [Spanish]. Madrid: LID.

Utesch, W. E. (1999). Book review of *The parental alienation syndrome. American Journal of Family Therapy, 27*(3):286.

Vallejo Orellana, Reyes, Fernando Sánchez-Barranco Vallejo, and Pablo Sánchez-Barranco Vallejo. (2004). Separación o divorcio: Trastornos psicológicos en los padres y los hijos [Separation or divorce: Psychological disorders in parents and children] [Spanish]. *Revista de la Asociación Española de Neuropsiquiatría*, (92):91–110.

ValueOptions. (2006). V-Codes: Relational problems. In: *ValueOptions provider handbook. www.valueoptions.com/providers/Handbook.htm*, accessed February 1, 2010.

Vanderheyden, Jean-Emile, Ed. (2008). *Approcher le divorce conflictuel [Approaching the Conflictual Divorce]* [French]. Malonne, Belgium: Feuilles Familiales Publishers.

Van Gijseghem, Hubert. (2002). Le Syndrome d'aliénation parentale [Parental alienation syndrome] [French]. *La Revue d'Action Juridique & Sociale*, (218):38–41.

Van Gijseghem, Hubert. (2004). L'aliénation parentale: Les principales controverses [Parental alienation: The principal controversies] [French]. *La Revue d'Action Juridique et Sociale*, (237):11–18.

Van Gijseghem, Hubert. (2005a). L'Aliénation parentale: Points controversés [Parental alienation: Controversies] [French]. *Divorce et Séparation*, (3):13–27.

Van Gijseghem, Hubert. (2005b). Les controverses entourant la notion de l'aliénation parentale [The controversies surrounding the notion of parental alienation] [French]. *Revue de Psychoéducation, 34*(1):119–29.

Van Gijseghem, Hubert. (2009). Belangrijkste controverses over ouderverstoting [Principal controversies regarding parental alienation] [Dutch]. In: *Verpasseerd Ouderschap [Boycotted Parenting]*, Ed. Joep Zander, pages 45–62. Deventer: Rela Publishing.

Van Gijseghem, Hubert. (2010). L'irréductible résistance au concept de l'aliénation parentale. [The ongoing resistance to the concept of parental alienation] [French]. *Revue de Psychoéducation, 39*(1):85–99.

Van Gijseghem, Hubert, and P. Lamontagne. (2008). L'aliénation parentale. Comment intervenir? [Parental alienation: How to intervene?] [French]. In: *Approcher le divorce conflictuel.[Approaches to High-conflict Divorce]*, Ed. J. E. Vanderheyden, pages 136–43. Namur, Belgium: Éditions Feuilles Familiales.

Van Horn, Patricia, and Betsy McAlister Groves. (2006). Children exposed to domestic violence: Making trauma-informed custody and visitation decisions. *Juvenile and Family Court Journal, 57*(1):51–60.

van Rooyen, Celest L., and Bala Mahendra. (2007). Parental alienation. In: *Psychology in Family and Child Law,* pages 61–66. Bristol, U.K.: Family Law.

Vassiliou, Despina. (2005). The Impact of the Legal System on Parental Alienation Syndrome. Dissertation, McGill University, Montreal.

Vassiliou, Despina, and Glenn F. Cartwright. (2001). The lost parents' perspective on parental alienation syndrome. *American Journal of Family Therapy, 29*(3):181–91.

Vestal, Anita. (1999). Mediation and parental alienation syndrome: Considerations for an intervention model. *Family & Conciliation Courts Review, 37*(4):487–503.

Volz, Jennifer. (2005). Das Elterliche Entfremdungssyndrom (PAS) [The Parental Alienation Syndrome (PAS)] [German]. Dissertation, Pädagogische Hochschule Karlsruhe, Karlsruhe, Germany.

Waldron, Kenneth H., and David E. Joanis. (1996). Understanding and collaboratively treating parental alienation syndrome. *American Journal of Family Law, 10*(3):121–33.

Walker, April J. (2006). The extreme consequence of parental alienation syndrome –The Richard Lohstroh case of a child driven to kill his father–Will courts move toward allowing children to use parental alienation syndrome as a defense to the crime of murder of their own parent? *Women's Rights Law Reporter, 27*(3):153–64.

Walker, Lenore E. A., Kristi L. Brantley, and Justin A. Rigsbee. (2004a). A critical analysis of parental alienation syndrome and its admissibility in the family court. *Journal of Child Custody, 1*(2):47–74.

Walker, Lenore E. A., Kristi L. Brantley, and Justin A. Rigsbee. (2004b). Response to Johnston and Kelly critique of PAS article. *Journal of Child Custody, 1*(4):91–97.

Wallerstein, Judith S. (1985). Children of divorce: Preliminary report of a ten-year follow-up of older children and adolescents. *Journal of the American Academy of Child Psychiatry, 24*(5)545–53.

Wallerstein, Judith S., and Sandra Blakeslee. (1989). *Second chances: Men, women, and children a decade after divorce.* New York: Ticknor & Fields.

Wallerstein, Judith S., and Sandra Blakeslee. (2003). *What about the kids? Raising your children before, during, and after divorce.* New York: Hyperion.

Wallerstein, Judith S., and Julia M. Lewis. (1998). The long-term impact of divorce on children: A first report from a 25-year study. *Family & Conciliation Courts Review, 36:*368–83.

Wallerstein, Judith S., Julia M. Lewis, and Sandra Blakeslee. (2000). *The unexpected legacy of divorce–The 25-year landmark study.* New York: Hyperion.

Wallerstein, Judith S., and Joan B. Kelly. (1976). The effects of parental divorce: Experiences of the child in later latency. *American Journal of Orthopsychiatry, 46:*256–69.

Wallerstein, Judith S., and Joan B. Kelly. (1980). *Surviving the breakup.* New York: Basic Books.

Walsh, Michael R., and J. Michael Bone. (1997). Parental alienation syndrome: An age-old custody problem. *Florida Bar Journal, 71*(6):93–96.

Wamboldt, Marianne Z., Frederick S. Wamboldt, Leslie Gavin, and Sandra McTaggart. (2001). A parent-child relationship scale derived from the child and adolescent psychiatric assessment (CAPA). *Journal of the American Academy of Child and Adolescent Psychiatry, 40*(8):945–53.

Ward, Peggy, and J. Campbell Harvey (1993). Family wars: The alienation of children. *New Hampshire Bar Journal, 34*(1):30–40.

Warshak, Richard A. (1999). Psychological syndromes: Parental alienation syndrome. In: *Expert Witness Manual,* Ed. R. Orsinger, pages 3:32:31–33:32:27. Austin, Texas: State Bar of Texas.

Warshak, Richard A. (2000). Remarriage as a trigger of parental alienation syndrome. *American Journal of Family Therapy, 28*(3):229–41.

Warshak, Richard A. (2001a). *Divorce poison: Protecting the parent-child bond from a vindictive ex.* New York: HarperCollins.

Warshak, Richard A. (2001b). Current controversies regarding parental alienation syndrome. *American Journal of Forensic Psychology, 19*(3):29–59.

Warshak, Richard A. (2002). Misdiagnosis of parental alienation syndrome. *American Journal of Forensic Psychology, 20*(2):31–52.

Warshak, Richard A. (2003a). Bringing sense to parental alienation: A look at the disputes and the evidence. *Family Law Quarterly, 37*(2):273–301.

Warshak, Richard A. (2003b). Payoffs and pitfalls of listening to children. *Family Relations, 52*(4):373–84.

Warshak, Richard A. (2005). Eltern-Kind-Entfremdung und Sozialwissenschaften–Sachlichkeit statt Polemik [Parent-child alienation and social science–Objectivity instead of polemics] [German]. *Zentralblatt für Jugendrecht, 92*(5):186–200.

Warshak, Richard A. (2006). Social science and parental alienation: Examining the disputes and the evidence. In Richard A. Gardner, S. Richard Sauber, and Demosthenes Lorandos (Eds.), *The international handbook of parental alienation syndrome: Conceptual, clinical and legal consideration,* pages 352–71. Springfield, Illinois: Charles C Thomas.

Warshak, Richard A. (2010a). Family Bridges: Using insights from social science to reconnect parents and alienated children. *Family Court Review, 48*(1)48–80.

Warshak, Richard A. (2010b). Alienating audiences from innovation: The perils of polemics, ideology, and innuendo. *Family Court Review, 48*(1)153–163.

Warshak, Richard A. (2010c). *Divorce poison: How to protect your family from bad-mouthing and brainwashing.* New York: HarperPaperbacks.

Warshak, Richard A., and Mark R. Otis. (2010). Helping alienated children with Family Bridges: Practice, research, and the pursuit of "humbition." *Family Court Review, 48*(1)91–97.

Watson, Andrew S. (1969). The children of Armageddon: Problems of custody following divorce. *Syracuse Law Review, 21*:55–86.

Webb, Eugene J., Donald T. Campbell, Richard D. Schwartz, and Lee Sechrest. (1966). *Unobtrusive measures: Nonreactive measures in the social science.* Chicago: Rand McNally.

Weigel, Daniel J., and Kimberly A. Donovan. (2006). Parental alienation syndrome: Diagnostic and triadic perspectives. *Family Journal, 14*(3):274–82.

Weintraub, Pamela., and Terry, Hillman. (2005). *Complete idiot's guide to surviving divorce* (3rd ed.). New York: Penguin Group.

Weir, Kirk. (2006). Clinical advice to courts on children's contact with their parents following parental separation. *Child and Adolescent Mental Health, 11*(1):40–46.

Weisbrodt, Franz. (2003). Möglichkeiten des Familienrichters, den Umgang des Trennungs-/Scheidungskindes mit beiden Eltern sicherzustellen [Enforcement of visitation and protection of family relationships with both parents for children of divorce by the court] [German]. In: *Das Parental Alienation Syndrom: Eine interdisziplinäre Herausforderung für scheidungsbegleitende Berufe,* Eds. Wilfrid von Boch-Galhau et al., pages 55–84. Berlin: Verlag für Wissenschaft und Bildung.

Weissman Herbert N. (1991), Forensic psychological examination of the child witness in cases of alleged sexual abuse. *American Journal of Orthopsychiatry, 61*(1):48–58.

Welter, Nicole. (2005). Vom Rambo-Jesus zu einer gut integrierten Männlichkeit [From Rambo-Jesus to well integrated masculinity] [German]. *Praxis der Kinderpsychologie und Kinderpsychiatrie, 54*(1):37–58.

Westman, Jack C., David W. Cline, William J. Swift, and Douglas A. Kramer. (1970). Role of child psychiatry in divorce. *Archives of General Psychiatry, 23*(5):416–20.

Willbourne, Caroline, and Lesley-Anne Cull. (1997). The emerging problem of parental alienation. *Family Law, 27*:807–08.

Williams, Frank S. (1990). Preventing Parentectomy Following Divorce. National Council for Children's Rights Annual Conference, Washington, D.C., October 20, 1990.

Williams, R. James. (2001). Should judges close the gate on PAS and PA? *Family Court Review, 39*(3):267–81.

Williams, Susan. (2006). Book review of *A Handbook of Divorce and Custody: Forensic, Developmental, and Clinical Perspectives. Journal of the American Academy of Child and Adolescent Psychiatry, 34*(1):136.

Wolchik, Sharlene A., and Paul Karoly, Eds. (1985). *Children of divorce: Empirical perspective on adjustment.* Dalton, Ohio: Gardner Press.

Wood, Cheri L. (1994). The parental alienation syndrome: A dangerous aura of reliability. *Loyola of Los Angeles Law Review, 27*(4):1367–415.

Worenklein, Abraham. (1992). Custody litigation and parental alienation. *International Journal of Psychology, 27*(3–4):226.

World Health Organization. (2007). *International statistical classification of diseases and related health problems* (10th ed.). Geneva: World Health Organization.

Xaxá, Igor Nazarovicz. (2008). A Síndrome De Alienação Parentale Eo Poder Judiciário [The parental alienation syndrome and the judiciary] [Portuguese]. Dissertation, Universidade Paulista–UNIP, Brazilia.

Zander, Joep, Ed. (2009). *Verpasseerd ouderschap [Parenting broken by PAS]* [Dutch]. Deventer, Netherlands: Relapublishing.

Zeitlin, Harry. (2007). Acrimonious contact disputes and so-called parental alienation syndrome: A model of understanding to assist with resolution. *Medico-legal Journal, 75*(Pt 4):143–49.

Zicavo Martínez, Nelson. (2008). La Alienación Parental y el Proceso de la Padrectomía [Parental alienation and the process of fatherectomy] [Spanish]. *Revista Cubana de Psicología* Commerative Edition (November 2008):57–62.

Zirogiannis, Lewis. (2001). Evidentiary issues with parental alienation syndrome. *Family Court Review, 39*(3):334–43.

NAME INDEX

A

Adams, K., 109, 180
Aguilar, J. M., vii, xxii, 72, 73
Ainsworth, M., 111, 112
Andre, K., vii
Andritzky, W., 64
Anthony, E. J., vii, xxii, 82
Arch Marin, M., vii, 74

B

Bakalář, E., vii, xxi, 59
Baker, A. J. L., viii, xxii, 39, 40, 87, 97, 117, 118, 179
Bala, N., 49, 50, 52, 80
Baldwin, Alec, 109, 180
Baris, M. A., 44, 119
Beach, S., 12
Beardslee, W. R., 84
Beeble, M., 87
Behrend, K., 66, 83
Benedek, E. P., 21, 82
Bensussan, Paul, viii, xxi, 61, 62
Bernet, A. C., viii, xxiii
Bernet, K. C., viii, xxiii
Bernet, W., xviii, xix, xxi, xxiii, 44, 45, 51, 87
Berns, S. S., 53, 54, 87
Bien, B. S., viii
Birchler-Hoop, U., 79
Birnbaum, Rachel, 49
Blackstone-Ford, J., 180
Blakeslee, S., 25, 111, 119
Boch-Galhau, W. v., viii, xxi, 52, 64, 65, 86, 113
Boerner, C., xxii
Bolaños, C., 74

Bone, J. M., viii, 46, 71
Bottinelli, J., 41
Bouza, J. M., 53
Bow, J. N., 42, 97, 98
Bowen, M., 89
Bowlby, J., 111, 112, 119
Boyan, S., 122
Brewer, M. B., 90, 91
Bricklin, B., viii, xxii, 31, 32
Brock, M. G., 50
Brockhausen, T., viii
Brögger, J., 70
Brownstone, H., 57
Bruch, C. S., 130, 131, 132, 133, 134
Bruck, M., 84
Burrill, J., 37
Buzzi, I., 67

C

Campbell, D. T., 23
Campbell, L. E. G., 28
Camps, A., 64, 66
Carey, K. M., 37
Cartié, M., 73, 74
Cartwright, G., 36, 43, 87, 113, 119
Cavedon, A., 67
Ceci, S. J., 83, 84
Chambers, A. J., ix, xxii
Chambers, P., 155, 156
Chrzanowski, C., 184
Clawar, S., 27, 28, 35
Cline, D., 20
Coca Vila, A., ix, 73
Colarossi, M., 41
Corrêa da Fonseca, P. M. P., 56

231

SUBJECT INDEX

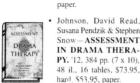

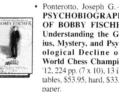

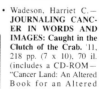

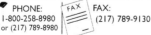